CMA® Skill Practice!

Certified Medical Assistant® Practice Test Questions

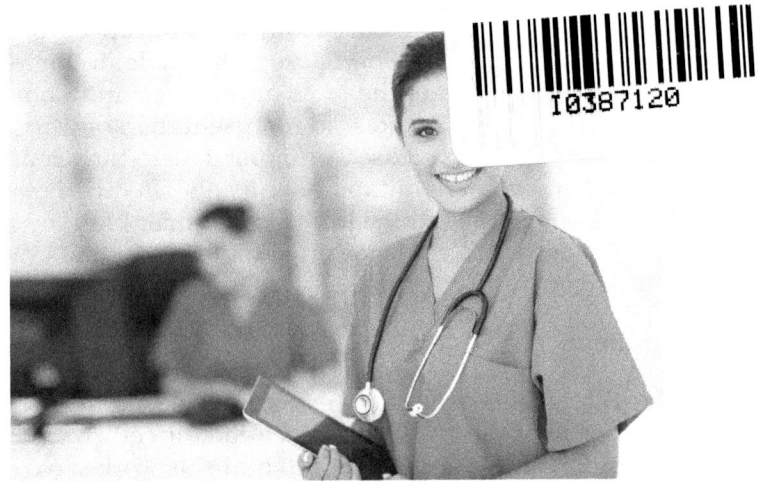

Published by

Complete TEST Preparation Inc.

Copyright © 2011 Complete Test Preparation Inc. ALL RIGHTS RESERVED.

No part of this book may be reproduced or transferred in any form or by any means, graphic, electronic, or mechanical, including photocopying, recording, web distribution, taping, or by any information storage retrieval system, without the written permission of the author.

Notice: Complete Test Preparation Inc. makes every reasonable effort to obtain from reliable sources accurate, complete, and timely information about the subjects covered in this book. Nevertheless, changes can be made in the tests or the administration of the tests at any time and Complete Test Preparation Inc. makes no representation or warranty of any kind, either expressed or implied as to the accuracy, timeliness, reliability, suitability or availability with respect to the information contained in this document for any purpose. Any reliance you place on such information is therefore strictly at your own risk.

Disclaimer

The author(s) shall not be liable for any loss incurred as a consequence of the use and application, directly or indirectly, of any information presented in this work. Sold with the understanding, the author is not engaged in rendering professional services or advice. If advice or expert assistance is required, the services of a competent professional should be sought.

Complete Test Preparation Inc. and the author(s) shall have neither liability nor responsibility to any person or entity with respect to any loss or damages arising form the information contained in this book.

The company, product and service names used in this publication are for identification purposes only. All trademarks and registered trademarks are the property of their respective owners. Complete Test Preparation Inc. is not affiliated with any educational institution. Use of a term in this book should not be regarded as affecting the validity of any trademark or service mark.

We strongly recommend that students check with exam providers for up-to-date information regarding test content.

CMA and Certified Medical Assistant are registered trademarks of the American Association of Medical Assistants, who are not involved in the production of, and do not endorse this book.

ISBN-13: 978-1-77245-054-5

Version 6.5 June 2015

Published by
Complete Test Preparation Inc.
921 Foul Bay Rd.
Victoria BC Canada V8S 4H9
Visit us on the web at http://www.test-preparation.ca
Printed in the USA

About Complete Test Preparation Inc.

Complete Test Preparation Inc. has been publishing high quality study materials since 2005. Thousands of students visit our websites every year, and thousands of students, teachers and parents all over the world have purchased our teaching materials, curriculum, study guides and practice tests.

Complete Test Preparation Inc. is committed to providing students with the best study materials and practice tests available on the market. Members of our team combine years of teaching experience, with experienced writers and editors, all with advanced degrees (Masters or higher).

Feedback

We Welcome your comments! You can email us (feedback@test-preparation.ca. and let us know what you think! We will carefully review your comments and may include them in future revisions.

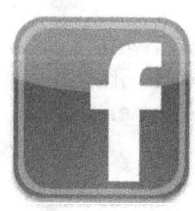

Find us on Facebook

www.facebook.com/CompleteTestPreparation

Contents

6	**Getting Started**	
	What is on the CMA®	6
8	**Practice Test Questions Set 1**	
	Answer Key	76
111	**Practice Test 2**	
	Answer Key	178
210	**Conclusion**	
211	**Multiple Choice Secrets!**	

Getting Started

CONGRATULATIONS! By deciding to take the Certified Medical Assistant Exam (CMA®), you have taken the first step toward a great future! Of course, there is no point in taking this important examination unless you intend to do your very best in order to earn the highest grade you possibly can. That means getting yourself organized and discovering the best approaches, methods and strategies to master the material. Yes, that will require real effort and dedication on your part but if you are willing to focus your energy and devote the study time necessary, before you know it you will be opening that letter of acceptance for the job of your dreams.

What is on the CMA®

The CMA® has six sections: Medical Terminology, Anatomy and Physiology, Communication Skills, Fundamental Writing Skills, Legal Issues and Legislation, and Insurance.

Part I – Medical Terminology
This section covers medical root, stems, prefixes and suffixes, common surgical procedures, diagnostic procedures and medical specialties.

Part II – Anatomy and Physiology
This section covers the functions, conditions and common diseases and issues with the different body systems.

Part III - Medical Legal and Ethical Issues and Legislation
This section covers medical legal issues, and important workplace and medical related legislation, including, Occupational Safety & Health (OSHA), Food & Drug Admin (FDA), Americans with Disabilities Act (ADA)

Part IV - Communication and Patient Education
This section covers basic communication skills such as, body language, listening skills, identifying needs, open and closed questions, active listening.

Part IV – Common Writing Skills
This section covers sentence structure, grammar and punctuation.

Part V – Insurance, Records and Bookkeeping
This section covers common office practice, accounting and bookkeeping, types of insurance and insurance codes.

Practice Test Questions Set 1

The questions below are not the same as you will find on the CMA® - that would be too easy! And nobody knows what the questions will be and they change all the time. Below are general questions that cover the same subject areas as the CMA®. So, while the format and exact wording of the questions may differ slightly, and change from year to year, if you can answer the questions below, you will have no problem with the CMA®.

For the best results, take these Practice Test Questions as if it were the real exam. Set aside time when you will not be disturbed, and a location that is quiet and free of distractions. Read the instructions carefully, read each question carefully, and answer to the best of your ability.

Use the bubble answer sheets provided. When you have completed the Practice Questions, check your answer against the Answer Key and read the explanation provided.

Do not attempt more than one set of practice test questions in one day. After completing the first practice test, wait two or three days before attempting the second set of questions.

Part I – Medical Terminology

1. Ⓐ Ⓑ Ⓒ Ⓓ
2. Ⓐ Ⓑ Ⓒ Ⓓ
3. Ⓐ Ⓑ Ⓒ Ⓓ
4. Ⓐ Ⓑ Ⓒ Ⓓ
5. Ⓐ Ⓑ Ⓒ Ⓓ
6. Ⓐ Ⓑ Ⓒ Ⓓ
7. Ⓐ Ⓑ Ⓒ Ⓓ
8. Ⓐ Ⓑ Ⓒ Ⓓ
9. Ⓐ Ⓑ Ⓒ Ⓓ
10. Ⓐ Ⓑ Ⓒ Ⓓ
11. Ⓐ Ⓑ Ⓒ Ⓓ
12. Ⓐ Ⓑ Ⓒ Ⓓ
13. Ⓐ Ⓑ Ⓒ Ⓓ
14. Ⓐ Ⓑ Ⓒ Ⓓ
15. Ⓐ Ⓑ Ⓒ Ⓓ
16. Ⓐ Ⓑ Ⓒ Ⓓ
17. Ⓐ Ⓑ Ⓒ Ⓓ
18. Ⓐ Ⓑ Ⓒ Ⓓ
19. Ⓐ Ⓑ Ⓒ Ⓓ
20. Ⓐ Ⓑ Ⓒ Ⓓ
21. Ⓐ Ⓑ Ⓒ Ⓓ
22. Ⓐ Ⓑ Ⓒ Ⓓ
23. Ⓐ Ⓑ Ⓒ Ⓓ
24. Ⓐ Ⓑ Ⓒ Ⓓ
25. Ⓐ Ⓑ Ⓒ Ⓓ
26. Ⓐ Ⓑ Ⓒ Ⓓ
27. Ⓐ Ⓑ Ⓒ Ⓓ
28. Ⓐ Ⓑ Ⓒ Ⓓ
29. Ⓐ Ⓑ Ⓒ Ⓓ
30. Ⓐ Ⓑ Ⓒ Ⓓ
31. Ⓐ Ⓑ Ⓒ Ⓓ
32. Ⓐ Ⓑ Ⓒ Ⓓ
33. Ⓐ Ⓑ Ⓒ Ⓓ
34. Ⓐ Ⓑ Ⓒ Ⓓ
35. Ⓐ Ⓑ Ⓒ Ⓓ
36. Ⓐ Ⓑ Ⓒ Ⓓ
37. Ⓐ Ⓑ Ⓒ Ⓓ
38. Ⓐ Ⓑ Ⓒ Ⓓ
39. Ⓐ Ⓑ Ⓒ Ⓓ
40. Ⓐ Ⓑ Ⓒ Ⓓ
41. Ⓐ Ⓑ Ⓒ Ⓓ
42. Ⓐ Ⓑ Ⓒ Ⓓ
43. Ⓐ Ⓑ Ⓒ Ⓓ
44. Ⓐ Ⓑ Ⓒ Ⓓ
45. Ⓐ Ⓑ Ⓒ Ⓓ
46. Ⓐ Ⓑ Ⓒ Ⓓ
47. Ⓐ Ⓑ Ⓒ Ⓓ
48. Ⓐ Ⓑ Ⓒ Ⓓ
49. Ⓐ Ⓑ Ⓒ Ⓓ
50. Ⓐ Ⓑ Ⓒ Ⓓ
51. Ⓐ Ⓑ Ⓒ Ⓓ
52. Ⓐ Ⓑ Ⓒ Ⓓ
53. Ⓐ Ⓑ Ⓒ Ⓓ
54. Ⓐ Ⓑ Ⓒ Ⓓ
55. Ⓐ Ⓑ Ⓒ Ⓓ
56. Ⓐ Ⓑ Ⓒ Ⓓ
57. Ⓐ Ⓑ Ⓒ Ⓓ
58. Ⓐ Ⓑ Ⓒ Ⓓ
59. Ⓐ Ⓑ Ⓒ Ⓓ
60. Ⓐ Ⓑ Ⓒ Ⓓ

Part II – Anatomy and Physiology

Part III – Medical Law, Ethics and Legislation

1. Ⓐ Ⓑ Ⓒ Ⓓ   11. Ⓐ Ⓑ Ⓒ Ⓓ   21. Ⓐ Ⓑ Ⓒ Ⓓ
2. Ⓐ Ⓑ Ⓒ Ⓓ   12. Ⓐ Ⓑ Ⓒ Ⓓ   22. Ⓐ Ⓑ Ⓒ Ⓓ
3. Ⓐ Ⓑ Ⓒ Ⓓ   13. Ⓐ Ⓑ Ⓒ Ⓓ   23. Ⓐ Ⓑ Ⓒ Ⓓ
4. Ⓐ Ⓑ Ⓒ Ⓓ   14. Ⓐ Ⓑ Ⓒ Ⓓ   24. Ⓐ Ⓑ Ⓒ Ⓓ
5. Ⓐ Ⓑ Ⓒ Ⓓ   15. Ⓐ Ⓑ Ⓒ Ⓓ   25. Ⓐ Ⓑ Ⓒ Ⓓ
6. Ⓐ Ⓑ Ⓒ Ⓓ   16. Ⓐ Ⓑ Ⓒ Ⓓ   26. Ⓐ Ⓑ Ⓒ Ⓓ
7. Ⓐ Ⓑ Ⓒ Ⓓ   17. Ⓐ Ⓑ Ⓒ Ⓓ   27. Ⓐ Ⓑ Ⓒ Ⓓ
8. Ⓐ Ⓑ Ⓒ Ⓓ   18. Ⓐ Ⓑ Ⓒ Ⓓ   28. Ⓐ Ⓑ Ⓒ Ⓓ
9. Ⓐ Ⓑ Ⓒ Ⓓ   19. Ⓐ Ⓑ Ⓒ Ⓓ   29. Ⓐ Ⓑ Ⓒ Ⓓ
10. Ⓐ Ⓑ Ⓒ Ⓓ   20. Ⓐ Ⓑ Ⓒ Ⓓ   30. Ⓐ Ⓑ Ⓒ Ⓓ

Part IV – Communication and Patient Education

1. Ⓐ Ⓑ Ⓒ Ⓓ   11. Ⓐ Ⓑ Ⓒ Ⓓ
2. Ⓐ Ⓑ Ⓒ Ⓓ   12. Ⓐ Ⓑ Ⓒ Ⓓ
3. Ⓐ Ⓑ Ⓒ Ⓓ   13. Ⓐ Ⓑ Ⓒ Ⓓ
4. Ⓐ Ⓑ Ⓒ Ⓓ   14. Ⓐ Ⓑ Ⓒ Ⓓ
5. Ⓐ Ⓑ Ⓒ Ⓓ   15. Ⓐ Ⓑ Ⓒ Ⓓ
6. Ⓐ Ⓑ Ⓒ Ⓓ   16. Ⓐ Ⓑ Ⓒ Ⓓ
7. Ⓐ Ⓑ Ⓒ Ⓓ   17. Ⓐ Ⓑ Ⓒ Ⓓ
8. Ⓐ Ⓑ Ⓒ Ⓓ   18. Ⓐ Ⓑ Ⓒ Ⓓ
9. Ⓐ Ⓑ Ⓒ Ⓓ   19. Ⓐ Ⓑ Ⓒ Ⓓ
10. Ⓐ Ⓑ Ⓒ Ⓓ   20. Ⓐ Ⓑ Ⓒ Ⓓ

Part V – Insurance, Records and Bookkeeping

1. Ⓐ Ⓑ Ⓒ Ⓓ 11. Ⓐ Ⓑ Ⓒ Ⓓ 21. Ⓐ Ⓑ Ⓒ Ⓓ
2. Ⓐ Ⓑ Ⓒ Ⓓ 12. Ⓐ Ⓑ Ⓒ Ⓓ 22. Ⓐ Ⓑ Ⓒ Ⓓ
3. Ⓐ Ⓑ Ⓒ Ⓓ 13. Ⓐ Ⓑ Ⓒ Ⓓ 23. Ⓐ Ⓑ Ⓒ Ⓓ
4. Ⓐ Ⓑ Ⓒ Ⓓ 14. Ⓐ Ⓑ Ⓒ Ⓓ 24. Ⓐ Ⓑ Ⓒ Ⓓ
5. Ⓐ Ⓑ Ⓒ Ⓓ 15. Ⓐ Ⓑ Ⓒ Ⓓ
6. Ⓐ Ⓑ Ⓒ Ⓓ 16. Ⓐ Ⓑ Ⓒ Ⓓ
7. Ⓐ Ⓑ Ⓒ Ⓓ 17. Ⓐ Ⓑ Ⓒ Ⓓ
8. Ⓐ Ⓑ Ⓒ Ⓓ 18. Ⓐ Ⓑ Ⓒ Ⓓ
9. Ⓐ Ⓑ Ⓒ Ⓓ 19. Ⓐ Ⓑ Ⓒ Ⓓ
10. Ⓐ Ⓑ Ⓒ Ⓓ 20. Ⓐ Ⓑ Ⓒ Ⓓ

Part VI – Fundamental Writing Skills

1. A B C D
2. A B C D
3. A B C D
4. A B C D
5. A B C D
6. A B C D
7. A B C D
8. A B C D
9. A B C D
10. A B C D
11. A B C D
12. A B C D
13. A B C D
14. A B C D
15. A B C D
16. A B C D
17. A B C D
18. A B C D
19. A B C D
20. A B C D
21. A B C D
22. A B C D
23. A B C D
24. A B C D
25. A B C D
26. A B C D
27. A B C D
28. A B C D
29. A B C D
30. A B C D
31. A B C D
32. A B C D
33. A B C D
34. A B C D
35. A B C D

Part I - Medical Terminology

1. Which, if any, of the following statements is false?

   a. Appendicitis is inflammation of the vermiform appendix.

   b. An appendectomy is a surgical procedure to remove that organ.

   c. Appendicitis may be acute, subacute, or chronic.

   d. Cathartics or enemas should be administered to prepare the patient for surgery.

2. A/an _____ is a procedure in which both the _____ _____ and some of the surrounding tissue are excised to eliminate cancer or to treat _____ or a/an _____.

   a. A radical prostatectomy is a procedure in which both the prostate gland and some of the surrounding tissue are excised to eliminate cancer or to treat benign prostatic hyperplasia or an enlarged prostate.

   b. A modified prostatectomy is a procedure in which both the prostate gland and some of the surrounding tissue are excised to eliminate cancer or to treat incontinence or an enlarged prostate.

   c. A radical vasectomy is a procedure in which both the prostate gland and some of the surrounding tissue are excised to eliminate cancer or to treat benign prostatic hyperplasia or an enlarged prostate.

   d. A hysterectomy is a procedure in which both the prostate gland and some of the surrounding tissue are excised to eliminate cancer or to treat benign prostatic hyperplasia or an enlarged prostate.

3. The _____ is a pear-shaped sac located near the right lobe of the liver that holds _____; a/an _____ is surgery to remove that organ.

   a. The pancreas is a pear-shaped sac located near the right lobe of the liver that holds bile; a/an pancreatectomy is surgery to remove that organ.

   b. The appendix is a pear-shaped sac located near the right lobe of the liver that holds bile; a/an cholecystectomy is surgery to remove that organ.

   c. The gall bladder is a pear-shaped sac located near the right lobe of the liver that holds bile; a/an appendectomy is surgery to remove that organ.

   d. The gall bladder is a pear-shaped sac located near the right lobe of the liver that holds bile; a/an cholecystectomy is surgery to remove that organ.

4. In cases of bladder stones or the removal of other tissue from the bladder, a/an _____ is performed by the insertion of a thin, lighted instrument through the urethra and into the bladder.

   a. Cystoscopy
   b. Arthroscopy
   c. Laparoscopy
   d. Appendectomy

5. A/an _____ allows a physician to examine the surfaces of the joints and surrounding tissues to diagnose joint complications, repair injuries, remove foreign bodies or monitor disease.

   a. Laminectomy
   b. Dilation
   c. Biopsy
   d. Arthroscopy

6. _____ is the most frequently performed surgery for the treatment of spinal stenosis; the procedure relieves pressure on the spinal cord caused by age-related changes in the spine.

    a. Carpal tunnel surgery

    b. Arthroscopy

    c. Decompressive laminectomy

    d. Lumbar puncture

7. Alternatives for the treatment of breast cancer include either _____ or _____ _____ or a _____ followed by radiation treatment.

    a. Alternatives for the treatment of breast cancer include either simple or modified complete mastectomy or a lumpectomy followed by radiation treatment.

    b. Alternatives for the treatment of breast cancer include either simple or complete mastectomy or a lumpectomy followed by radiation treatment.

    c. Alternatives for the treatment of breast cancer include either simple or radical mastectomy or a biopsy followed by radiation treatment.

    d. Alternatives for the treatment of breast cancer include either simple or modified radical lumpectomy or a mastectomy followed by radiation treatment.

8. Which, if any, of the following statements about bypass surgery is true?

    a. Bypass surgery is frequently performed the patient is experiencing angina.

    b. It is also done in cases of coronary artery disease when plaque has built up in the arteries.

    c. Bypass surgery provide an alternate route for blood flow if a vital artery has become obstructed.

    d. All of the above are true.

9. _____ are a group of tests that are performed together to detect, evaluate, and monitor disease or damage. This procedure determines levels of albumin and bilirubin, among others.

   a. A standard liver panel
   b. A complete blood count
   c. Cerebrospinal fluid analysis
   d. Biopsy

10. A/an _____ refers to the test usually used to screen for HIV infection.

   a. A standard liver panel
   b. Cisternography
   c. Electroencephalography
   d. Enzyme Linked Immunosorbent Assay (ELISA.

11. Which, of any, of the following statements about ultrasound scanning is false?

   a. Ultrasound imaging uses high-frequency sound waves to obtain internal body images.
   b. A neurosonography is an ultrasound of the brain and spinal column that can diagnose strokes and brain tumors.
   c. Ultrasound imaging is less effective than x-rays at revealing soft tissue damage such as torn ligaments, muscles and tendons.
   d. Painful inflammatory processes can be identified through the use of ultrasound imagery.

12. A/an _____ provides information about the number and percentage of red and white blood cells and platelets present. Because abnormally high or low counts are indicative of many types of disease, this test is one of the most commonly performed blood tests in medicine.

    a. Blood culture

    b. Complete blood count (CBC.

    c. Glucose tolerance test

    d. Chorionic villus sampling (CVS)

13. Testing for genetic defects is possible through the use of _____, usually done at 14 to 16 weeks of pregnancy.

    a. Amniocentesis

    b. Chorionic villus sampling (CVS)

    c. Ultrasound imaging

    d. Biopsy

14. Which, if any, of the following statements about neurological examinations are true?

    a. Mental function is determined through mental status exams (MSE) and a global assessment of higher functioning.

    b. Neurological cerebellar testing modalities include dysmetria (finger-to-nose) and ataxia to determine problems with gait.

    c. Examinations are aimed at ruling out the most clinically significant causes and diagnosing the most likely causes.

    d. All of the above are true.

15. Which diagnostic procedure used equipment to develop an image clearly displaying areas of differing density and composition?

    a. Ultrasound imaging

    b. Radiography

    c. Electroencephalography

    d. Fluoroscopy

16. A _____ is a microbiological culture of blood used to detect infections such as bacteria and septicemia.

    a. Complete blood count

    b. Amniocentesis

    c. Blood culture

    d. Chorionic villus sampling (CVS)

17. _____ is a branch of medicine that deals with the _____ system and its production of hormones, which coordinate metabolism, respiration, and excretion, among others. Medical professionals in this field treat persons with diabetes, thyroid diseases, cholesterol disorders, and metabolic disorders.

    a. Endocrinology, endocrine

    b. Gastroenterology, digestive

    c. Hepatology, digestive

    d. Urology

18. Which, if any, of the following statements about geriatrics are false?

    a. Geriatrics is a branch of medicine in which the focus is health care for the aging population.

    b. Geriatrics differs from gerontology, which is the study of the aging process itself.

    c. A geriatrician's practice is limited to persons over the age of 65.

    d. None of the above.

19. _____ is the medical specialty involved in the study of the liver, gallbladder, biliary tree, and pancreas and diseases such as viral hepatitis and alcohol-related conditions.

    a. Hepatology
    b. Immunology
    c. Oncology
    d. Nephrology

20. _____ surgeons use their skills to correct diseases, defects and injuries in the head, neck, face, jaws and the hard and soft tissues of the oral and facial region.

    a. Ear, nose and throat (ENT)
    b. Orthopedic
    c. Reconstructive
    d. Oral and Maxillofacial

21. Which, if any, of the following statements concerning palliative medicine are false?

    a. Palliative medicine is another name for hospice care.

    b. Palliative medicine addresses the needs of patients in all stages of a disease or illness, including those undergoing treatment for curable diseases and those living with chronic illness.

    c. It is a branch of medicine that is focused on both relieving and preventing the suffering of patients.

    d. Palliative medicine relies on input from many sources, including nurses, pharmacists, chaplains and psychologists, among others.

22. Patients who have been diagnosed with acute renal failure, chronic kidney disease, hematuria, kidney stones or hypertension are usually referred to _____.

    a. Pathologists

    b. Hepatologists

    c. Nephrologists

    d. Internists

23. The practice of _____ is concerned with the diagnosis of cancer as well as cancer therapies such as surgery, chemotherapy and radiotherapy as well as follow-up of such cases and palliative care for patients in the terminal stages of cancer.

    a. Pathology

    b. Internal medicine

    c. Oncology

    d. Physical medicine

24. _____ is a branch of medicine that addresses the causes (etiology), mechanisms of development (pathogenesis), structural alterations of cells (morphologic changes), and the consequences of those changes (clinical manifestations or diseases).

    a. Internal medicine
    b. Pathology
    c. Nephrology
    d. None of the above.

25. The greek root -pepsia means

    a. disease.
    b. digestion.
    c. respiration.
    d. vision.

26. The Greek root -apathy means,

    a. disease.
    b. viruses.
    c. bacteria.
    d. fever.

27. The Latin root abdomin- means related to,

    a. the appendix.
    b. the abdomen area.
    c. the larynx.
    d. the lungs.

28. The Greek and Latin root aort means related to

    a. the arteries.

    b. the arms.

    c. the aorta.

    d. the anvil.

29. The Greek root brachi means related to

    a. the arm.

    b. the back.

    c. the mouth.

    d. the leg.

30. Which Greek root means artery?

    a. Arto-

    b. Artra-

    c. Arteri-

    d. Arturi-

31. Which Latin root means back?

    a. Spina-

    b. Dors-

    c. Backial-

    d. Cyst-

32. The Latin root allic- means relating to

    a. the calf.

    b. the little toe.

    c. the big toe.

    d. the ankle.

33. The Greek root cyst(o)- means relating to

   a. the bladder.
   b. the blood.
   c. the spine.
   d. the brain.

34. The Greek root hemat- means relating to

   a. the head.
   b. the heart.
   c. the blood.
   d. the lungs.

35. What Greek root means relating to blood clots?

   a. Thrum(o)-
   b. Angio-
   c. Somat-
   d. Cysto-

36. What Greek root means relating to the blood vessels?

   a. Ante-
   b. Amphi-
   c. Hemo-
   d. Angio-

37. What Greek root means relating to the chest?

   a. Masto-
   b. Stetho-
   c. Somat-
   d. Aden-

38. What Latin root means relating to the ear?

   a. Video-
   b. Osteo-
   c. Aur-
   d. Lipo-

39. The Greek root ophthalmo- means relating to

   a. the ears.
   b. the eyes.
   c. the nose.
   d. the heart.

40. The Greek root lipo- means relating to

   a. the fat.
   b. the eyes.
   c. the abdomen.
   d. the heart.

41. The Latin root digit- means relating to

   a. the eye.
   b. the toe.
   c. the finger.
   d. the face.

42. The Latin root manu- means relating to

   a. the foot.
   b. the hand.
   c. the eye.
   d. the face.

43. The Greek root cardi- means relating to

　a. the heart.
　b. the lungs.
　c. the head.
　d. the feet.

44. The Greek root entero- means relating to

　a. the heart.
　b. the intestine.
　c. the blood.
　d. the face.

45. The Latin root ren- means relating to

　a. the intestines.
　b. the bladder.
　c. the kidney.
　d. the appendix.

46. The Greek root trachel means relating to

　a. the neck.
　b. the mouth.
　c. the eyes.
　d. the spine.

47. The Greek root neuro- means relating to

　a. the arteries.
　b. the veins.
　c. the nerves.
　d. the muscles

48. The Greek root medi- in anatomy or other areas, means

    a. the top.

    b. the middle.

    c. the bottom.

    d. the entire being.

49. The Latin root equi, in anatomy or other areas, means

    a. equal.

    b. greater than.

    c. less than.

    d. the middle of something.

50. The Latin prefix ab-, in a medical context, means

    a. toward.

    b. away from.

    c. up from the ground.

    d. down from above.

51. The Greek prefix aesthesio, in a medical context, means

    a. sleep.

    b. painlessness.

    c. sensation.

    d. balance.

52. The Greek prefix bio-, in a medical context, means

    a. life.

    b. story.

    c. image.

    d. sound.

53. The Latin prefix capit-, in a medical context, means

   a. Heart.
   b. Breath / air.
   c. Torso.
   d. Head.

54. The Latin prefix carp-, in a medical context, means

   a. the wrist.
   b. the fingers.
   c. the nerves.
   d. the heart.

55. The Greek prefix cata-, in a medical context, means

   a. up or over.
   b. down or under.
   c. up and down.
   d. over and under.

56. The Latin prefix dis-, in a medical context, means

   a. putting something together.
   b. shutting something.
   c. taking something apart or separating.
   d. removing something.

57. The Greek prefix endo-, in a medical context, means

   a. outside of something.
   b. inside or within.
   c. around something.
   d. under.

58. The Greek prefix exo-, in a medical context, means

    a. something outside another.

    b. something inside another.

    c. something that lives off the body of another.

    d. something that an x-ray cannot penetrate.

59. The prefix fibro-, in a medical context, means

    a. vitamins.

    b. minerals.

    c. fiber.

    d. organic.

60. The prefix filli-, in a medical context, means

    a. hair-like or fine.

    b. organized.

    c. pertaining to the fingernails.

    d. contagious.

Part II – Anatomy & Physiology

1. Anatomy breaks the human abdomen down into segments called _____.

    a. regions

    b. districts

    c. quadrants

    d. areas

Practice Test Questions Set 1

2. The quadrant that is largely responsible for digestion is _____.

    a. left upper
    b. right upper
    c. right left
    d. left lower

3. The body organ that is NOT located within the Right Upper Quadrant is _____.

    a. liver
    b. gall bladder
    c. duodenum
    d. sigmoid colon

4. The organ that IS located in the Right Lower Quadrant is _____

    a. appendix
    b. heart
    c. left lung
    d. trachea

5. One reason that medical professionals should know the names and locations of the Quadrant is _____.

    a. to keep the patient's condition a secret from him.
    b. to communicate about patients' conditions with other doctors and medical professionals.
    c. for insurance purposes.
    d. not knowing the quadrants almost always results in death for the patient.

6. The stomach and colon are both in the _____.

    a. left upper quadrant

    b. right upper quadrant

    c. right lower quadrant

    d. left lower quadrant

7. Commonly used abbreviations for the Quadrants of the abdomen are _____.

    a. QUR, QUL, QLR, QLL

    b. ABC, DEF, GHI, JKL

    c. RUQ, LUQ, RLQ, LLQ

    d. RR, LL, QQ, RQ

8. The intestines are located in _____.

    a. LUQ

    b. LLQ

    c. RLQ

    d. All of the above

9. The stomach is located in _____.

    a. LLQ

    b. LUQ

    c. RUQ

    d. RLQ

10. The gallbladder is located in _____.

    a. RUQ

    b. LUQ

    c. LLQ

    d. RLQ

11. An example of human homeostasis is _____.

   a. metabolism
   b. adrenalin
   c. hormones
   d. fluid balance

12. Human homeostasis is the ability of the body to regulate its _____ in response to fluctuations in the environment outside the body.

   a. inner environment
   b. outer environment
   c. temperature
   d. metabolism

13. The amount of energy / calories that your body requires to maintain itself is known as _____.

   a. temperature
   b. fluid balance
   c. botulism
   d. metabolism

14. An example of a person whose metabolism has lowered is _____.

   a. a woman who is in her teens and quite athletic
   b. a man who is past 30 and whose body is losing muscle.
   c. a man who is past 30 and works out daily.
   d. a man who is past 30 and eats a low-fat diet.

15. An example of something that increases a person's metabolism is _____.

    a. aerobic exercise

    b. mental exercise

    c. eating a fatty diet

    d. reading

16. Fluid balance might be negatively impacted when the _____ fail.

    a. kidneys

    b. ears

    c. nose

    d. legs

17. Fluid balance is important, because _____ comprises about 60-70% of a person's weight.

    a. calcium

    b. water

    c. iron

    d. bone

18. As a person moves from adolescence to later adulthood, his metabolism _____.

    a. begins to get higher

    b. begins to get lower.

    c. stabilizes

    d. fluctuates wildly

19. "Met" refers to _____.

    a. mitosis

    b. the person's heart rate

    c. the person's blood pressure

    d. the person's metabolic rate.

20. Fluid balance is important, because the human body loses water every day through urination, perspiration, feces, and _____.

    a. breathing

    b. resting

    c. meditating

    d. outbursts of temper

21. The smallest unit of life in our bodies is the _____.

    a. atom

    b. molecule

    c. proton

    d. cell

22. One of the functions of the cell membrane is to _____.

    a. divide into other cells.

    b. control what moves into and out of the cell.

    c. fight infection.

    d. trap bacteria.

23. The process of a larger cell dividing into two or more smaller cells is _____.

    a. cell division.

    b. cell multiplication.

    c. mitosis.

    d. metabolism.

24. Prophase, metaphase, anaphase, and telophase are all phases of _____.

    a. cell division.

    b. infection.

    c. mitosis.

    d. adrenaline.

25. Mitosis is a scientific term that, in layman's terms, just means

    a. cellular disease.

    b. nuclear cell division (division of the cell nucleus).

    c. infection.

    d. atomic fusion.

26. The stage of mitosis in which the chromatin condenses and becomes a chromosome is _____.

    a. prophase

    b. metaphase

    c. anaphase

    d. telophase

27. The stage of mitosis in which the chromosomes begin to align is _____.

    a. prophase
    b. metaphase
    c. anaphase
    d. telophase

28. The stage of mitosis in which the paired chromosomes separate, each going to an opposite pole of the cell, is _____.

    a. metaphase
    b. prophase
    c. anaphase
    d. anaphase

29. The stage of mitosis in which the two chromosomes are cordoned into new nuclei within the daughter cells is _____.

    a. metaphase
    b. prophase
    c. anaphase
    d. telophase

30. Squamous, cuboidal and columnar are three kinds of what kind of cell tissue?

    a. epidermis
    b. epithelial tissue
    c. nerve tissue
    d. muscle tissue

31. An important function of epithelial tissue is _____.

    a. to strengthen the muscles.
    b. acting as a protective barrier for the human body.
    c. protect the nerves.
    d. nonexistent. it has no known function.

32. An important function of connective tissue is _____.

    a. acting as a protective barrier for the human body.
    b. protect the muscles.
    c. storage of energy.
    d. strengthen the nerves.

33. Muscle tissue has the ability to _____, bringing out movement and the ability to work.

    a. divide and conquer.
    b. replicate at will.
    c. relax and contract.
    d. sleep.

34. Nervous tissue is specialized to _____.

    a. do work.
    b. protect the body.
    c. teach the person to relax.
    d. react to stimuli.

35. Nerve tissue is made up of cells known as _____.

    a. neurons.
    b. protons
    c. molecules
    d. atoms

36. The bodily organ system, which protects the person's body from damage, is the _____ system.

   a. circulatory
   b. musculoskeletal
   c. integumentary
   d. digestive

37. The integumentary system comprises the _____ and its various appendages.

   a. skeleton
   b. brain
   c. skin
   d. heart

38. An example of appendages contained within the integumentary system are / is _____.

   a. lungs
   b. hair and nails
   c. nostrils
   d. ears

39. In addition to protecting the body, an example of a benefit of the integumentary system is its function of _____.

   a. circulating blood.
   b. digesting food.
   c. processing information.
   d. regulating temperature.

40. How many layers of skin are contained within the human integumentary system (skin)?

    a. one
    b. two
    c. three
    d. four

41. The names of the three layers of skin are,

    a. proton, neuron, nucleus.
    b. epidural, mitochondria, chromosome
    c. inner, outer, local
    d. epidermis, dermis and sub dermis.

42. Which sub-layer of skin gives it flexibility?

    a. the dermis
    b. epidermis
    c. subdermis
    d. dermatology

43. An example of a minor ailment of the integumentary system is _____.

    a. skin cancer
    b. acne
    c. common cold
    d. flu

44. An example of a serious ailment of the integumentary system is _____.

    a. acne

    b. skin cancer

    c. heart disease

    d. high blood pressure

45. Which body system is comprised mostly of bones?

    a. respiratory

    b. endocrine

    c. musculoskeletal

    d. integumentary

46. Joints are an example of what within the musculoskeletal system?

    a. bone tissue

    b. connective tissue

    c. muscles

    d. nerves

47. One of the primary purposes of the musculoskeletal system is

    a. providing stability to the body.

    b. distributing blood.

    c. providing infection control.

    d. eliminating waste.

48. Another primary purpose of the musculoskeletal system is

    a. moving oxygen.

    b. cleansing the blood stream.

    c. relaxing the mind.

    d. providing form for the body

49. What makes it sometimes difficult to diagnose an ailment within the musculoskeletal system?

    a. bones resist x-rays.

    b. there are no diseases associated with the musculoskeletal system.

    c. its close proximity to other organs within the body.

    d. its distant proximity away from other organs within the body.

50. What is cartilage?

    a. a flexible, connective tissue that keeps bones from rubbing against each other.

    b. the material that comprises the brain.

    c. a part of human blood responsible for fighting infection.

    d. another name for the femur.

Part III – Medical Ethics, Law and Legislation

1. _____ refers to the behaviors the medical professionals with moral integrity are expected to exhibit.

    a. Courtesy

    b. Mores

    c. Customs

    d. Medical ethics

2. The three issues that determine an incident of battery are:

    a. The patient has been given false information about a treatment.

    b. The patient is judged incompetent to consent to treatment and has received improper care.

    c. Care that the patient has refused is forced upon them without court authorization.

    d. All of the above

3. The four major principles of medical ethics are:

    a. Autonomy, beneficence, non-malfeasance and justice

    b. Privacy, autonomy, beneficence and justice

    c. Autonomy, beneficence, universality and justice

    d. Autonomy, beneficence, non-malfeasance and morality

4. The definition of a double effect does not state that:

   a. A double effect is a byproduct of non-malfeasance

   b. The action being considered is in itself either morally good or morally indifferent.

   c. There was no direct intention to cause harm.

   d. The beneficial result must be disproportionate to the harm caused by the action.

5. Which of these statements about the AAMA standards of practice is/are false?

   a. Only duly licensed physicians/dentists are required to report any knowledge of professional abuse to the appropriate authorities.

   b. As an AMT professional, you must place the welfare of the patient above all other considerations.

   c. The judgment of the attending physician/dentist shall be protected and valued, no matter what the circumstances.

   d. a. & c.

6. _____ is an ethical principle that states that communication between a patient and a provider must remain private.

   a. Autonomy

   b. Honesty

   c. Consent

   d. Confidentiality

7. _____ is the major principle of medical ethics that states that physicians and other medical professionals must act in the best interest of the patient.

   a. Justice
   b. Autonomy
   c. Non-malfeasance
   d. Beneficence

8. The principles of _____ and _____ must be balanced to be certain that any risks involved in medical treatment or procedures is outweighed by the benefit to the patient.

   a. Autonomy and privacy
   b. Dignity and justice
   c. Beneficence and non-malfeasance
   d. Ethics and beneficence

9. _____ is the ethical principle most applicable to the highly publicized issue of universal healthcare.

   a. Justice
   b. Autonomy
   c. Non-malfeasance
   d. Beneficence

10. A _____ system is a process by which treatment is prioritized based on needed personnel and those who are most critically ill or injured.

    a. Disaster
    b. Quarantine
    c. Pandemic
    d. Triage

11. A patient's agreement to treatment based on a clear understanding of their condition and all possible consequences of treatment is a/an _____.

   a. Full disclosure

   b. Legal standard

   c. Logical decision

   d. Informed consent

12. Some exceptions to the rule of informed consent are:

   a. Prior to a common procedure with little risk such as a blood test or in an emergency, life-threatening situation

   b. There are no exceptions to the rule; informed consent must always be obtained prior to treatment.

   c. The patient is a minor.

   d. The patient is suffering advanced dementia.

13. Before a patient exercises their right to refusal of treatment, they must be informed about:

   a. The diagnosis and prognosis of their medical condition

   b. Available alternative treatments and the risks and benefits of those options

   c. The risk and probable outcome of no intervention

   d. All of the above

14. Under certain conditions, a person must submit to _____ treatment, which is medical care or testing without their permission.

   a. Legally mandated

   b. Emergency exception

   c. Life saving

   d. Doctor ordered

15. The situations in which patients must submit to legally mandated treatments include:

    a. The patient has been judged incompetent and has been appointed a guardian.

    b. The patient has been involuntarily confined to a mental institution.

    c. A court has ordered treatment under the authority of public health laws.

    d. All of the above

16. A _____ is an exception to the requirement of informed consent and allows the withholding of information from a patient if such information would cause psychological damage and therefore endanger their physical well-being.

    a. Malpractice suit

    b. Therapeutic exception

    c. Mandated treatment

    d. Autonomy exception

17. Which of the following statements about medical malpractice is false?

    a. Medical malpractice occurs when a negligent act or omission by a doctor or other medical professional results in damage or harm to a patient.

    b. A medical malpractice suit can be filed any time that patient consent was not obtained prior to treatment.

    c. Negligence may involve an error in diagnosis, treatment, or illness management.

    d. A medical malpractice case can also be filed against a hospital for improper care or inadequate training.

18. Which of the following statements about torts is/are false?

    a. Torts are personal civil injuries that reside outside of a contractual relationship.

    b. Torts can be intentional, such as fraud, assault, etc.

    c. Torts result in criminal trials that assess guilt or innocence.

    d. Torts can be unintentional, such as negligence or malpractice.

19. A(n) _____ _____ is a legal document filed in advance by a patient which details their wishes in the event that they are incapacitated.

    a. Last will and testament

    b. Beneficiary list

    c. Advance directive

    d. Funeral plan

20. Which if any of the following statements about living wills is true?

    a. They state the type of care a patient does or does not want to receive at the end of their life.

    b. They are documents in which the patient chooses a surrogate who can make healthcare decisions in the event that they are incapacitated.

    c. They demand that no extraordinary measures such as CPR, are used in an effort to revive the patient.

    d. All of the above.

21. What are the two types of advance directives?

    a. A durable power of attorney and a DNR order

    b. A funeral plan and a living will

    c. A life insurance policy and a durable power of attorney

    d. A living will and a durable power of attorney

22. In addition to state laws, _____ is the law that governs the donation of organs and tissues.

    a. The Uniform Anatomical Gift Act

    b. The Americans with Disabilities Act

    c. The Organ Procurement and Use Act

    d. There is no law; organ donation is a civil matter between the hospital and a patient's next of kin.

23. While _____ is a mistake or a failure to be careful, _____ includes wrongful conduct by a professional or a failure to meet standards of care that results in harm to another person.

    a. While malpractice is a mistake or a failure to be careful, negligence includes wrongful conduct by a professional or a failure to meet standards of care that results in harm to another person.

    b. While negligence is a mistake or a failure to be careful, malpractice includes wrongful conduct by a professional or a failure to meet standards of care that results in harm to another person.

    c. While substandard behavior is a mistake or a failure to be careful, malpractice includes wrongful conduct by a professional or a failure to meet standards of care that results in harm to another person.

    d. While an intentional tort is a mistake or a failure to be careful, malfeasance includes wrongful conduct by a professional or a failure to meet standards of care that results in harm to another person.

24. What conditions usually preclude organ or tissue donation?

    a. Advanced age and metastatic cancer

    b. A history of hepatitis, HIV or AIDS

    c. Sepsis

    d. All of the above

25. In _____, the brain no longer functions organically and the patient is kept alive through the use of a ventilator. When a patient's cerebrum is dead and they are unconscious, cannot think or reason, but may still be breathing, they have experienced _____.

    a. In higher brain death, the brain no longer functions organically and the patient is kept alive through the use of a ventilator. When a patient's cerebrum is dead and they are unconscious, cannot think or reason, but may still be breathing, they have experienced whole brain death.

    b. In whole brain death, the brain no longer functions organically and the patient is kept alive through the use of a ventilator. When a patient's cerebrum is dead and they are unconscious, cannot think or reason, but may still be breathing, they have experienced partial brain death.

    c. In whole brain death, the brain no longer functions organically and the patient is kept alive through the use of a ventilator. When a patient's cerebrum is dead and they are unconscious, cannot think or reason, but may still be breathing, they have experienced higher brain death.

    d. In brain stem death, the brain no longer functions organically and the patient is kept alive through the use of a ventilator. When a patient's cerebrum is dead and they are unconscious, cannot think or reason, but may still be breathing, they have experienced cerebrum brain death.

26. What does OSHA stand for?

a. Oxford Safety and Humanities Administration.

b. Occupational Sales and Office Hazards Administration.

c. Occupational Safety and Health Administration.

d. Occupational Super Health Agency.

27. What is OSHA's chief function / purpose?

a. Overseeing private sector workplaces to prevent possible dangers or hazards that could affect the workers.

b. Monitoring gas leaks in government buildings.

c. Observing the ocean for dangerous storms.

d. Monitoring the deterioration of the Ozone Layer.

28. Which of the following is an example of a time when OSHA might initiate an inspection?

a. When there is a jar that was broken on a supermarket floor.

b. When a dangerous accident on the road has closed down traffic.

c. When workers have complained about an ongoing gas leak at the worksite.

d. When workers complain about inadequate pay.

29. Which of the following is true regarding an employer's compliance with OSHA guidelines?

a. OSHA demands that all employers comply with their final rules published under the 1970 Occupational Safety and Health Act. *

b. Compliance is completely voluntary.

c. Compliance is voluntary for small businesses with fewer than 100 worker but required at all other work places.

d. Compliance depends on the amount of money that the employer pays in health benefits.

30. What does FDA stand for?

a. Food and Drug Administration.

b. Federal Drug Agency.

c. Food Domain Agency.

d. Feeding Diabetic Americans.

Part IV – Communication and Patient Education

1. When communicating with another person, _____ is/are used to emphasize an important point, _____ can indicate either great interest or boredom, and _____ can express encouragement or empathy.

    a. When communicating with another person, gestures are used to emphasize an important point, posture can indicate either great interest or boredom, and touch can express encouragement or empathy.

    b. When communicating with another person, touch is used to emphasize an important point, posture can indicate either great interest or boredom, and gestures can express encouragement or empathy.

    c. When communicating with another person, posture is used to emphasize an important point, gestures can indicate either great interest or boredom, and touch can express encouragement or empathy.

    d. When communicating with another person, gestures are used to emphasize an important point, touch can indicate either great interest or boredom, and posture can express encouragement or empathy.

2. A person who is _____ may indicate the desire to place an unconscious barrier between themselves and others.

    a. Avoiding eye contact

    b. Yawning widely

    c. Making wild gestures

    d. Crossing their arms across their chest

3. Which, if any, of the following statements about eye contact are false?

   a. Consistent eye contact can indicate a positive reaction to a speaker.

   b. Consistent eye contact can indicate a lack of trust in the speaker.

   c. The use of eye contact may be dependent on the culture of the listener.

   d. None of these statements are false.

4. _____ is a technique used to put people at ease.

   a. Speaking softly
   b. Making eye contact
   c. Mirroring body language
   d. Leaning forward

5. Which, if any, of these statements about body language are false?

   a. Everyone uses some form of body language to communicate.

   b. Interpretations of body language are universal to all cultures.

   c. The study of body language is called kinetic interpretation.

   d. Indications of emotion such as smiling when happy are universal.

6. _____ can signal a lack of interest or an unfriendly attitude and can make therapeutic communication difficult to achieve.

   a. Eye contact
   b. Questioning
   c. Empathy
   d. Nonverbal communication

7. If a patient asks a question that is beyond the scope of your practice, the best response would be to:

    a. Make your best guess based on what you know.

    b. Tell the patient that you will find them the correct answer.

    c. Change the subject.

    d. Give them a book on the subject.

8. _____ is an important communication technique in which phrases such as "go on," please continue," and "tell me more" are used to encourage the patient.

    a. Facilitation

    b. Amplification

    c. Reflection

    d. Mirroring

9. _____ involves repeating something the patient just said to gain more specific information and to show that you are paying attention.

    a. Facilitation

    b. Reflection

    c. Mirroring

    d. None of the above

10. What are the two goals of the technique of summarization?

    a. To ensure that the information that you've collected is accurate and complete and to signal the end of the interview

    b. To obtain more specific information and to show that you are paying attention

    c. To gain the patient's trust and to obtain more specific information

    d. To make the interview as short as possible and to follow the rules as determined by the HMO.

11. _____ is restating something that a patient has said, usually in fewer words and with emphasis on the main points of their statement.

    a. Attending

    b. Paraphrasing

    c. Clarifying

    d. Perception checking

12. When _____ is used in active listening, it demonstrates that you understand the patient's experience and allows them to evaluate their feeling by hearing them expressed by someone else.

    a. Paraphrasing

    b. Summarization

    c. Clarifying

    d. Primary empathy

13. The steps to attentive listening include:

    a. Maintaining eye contact and facing the person squarely

    b. Sitting up straight and maintaining eye contact

    c. Taking careful notes and leaning toward the speaker

    d. Relaxing in your seat and slightly averting your eyes

14. Facial expression, posture and tone of voice are elements of _____.

    a. Open-ended questions

    b. Nonverbal communication

    c. Orientation process

    d. Good manners

15. **Which, if any, of the following statements about nonverbal communication are true?**

   a. Nonverbal communications are less reliable that verbal communication

   b. Nonverbal communications remain the same, regardless of ethnicity or culture.

   c. Nonverbal communications always send a clear message.

   d. Nonverbal communications can emphasize or contradict verbal messages.

16. _____ **are used to obtain the most complete information available.**

   a. Questionnaires and surveys

   b. Admission forms

   c. Open-ended questions

   d. Interviews

17. **Which, if any, of the following statements is false?**

   a. An interviewer should never ask close-ended questions.

   b. A close-ended question is one that can be answered "yes" or "no."

   c. An example of a close-ended question would be "Have you been having headaches for a long time?"

   d. A close-ended question verifies information already obtained.

18. _____ **provides encourages the patient to continue talking without indicating agreement or disagreement.**

   a. Smiling

   b. Leaning forward

   c. Nodding

   d. Paraphrasing

19. Using phrases that address a person's feelings, such as "You must be worried about your headaches," demonstrates _____.

   a. Empathy
   b. Interest
   c. Acceptance
   d. Recognition

20. _____ can be an effective way to communicate with children.

   a. Telling stories
   b. Reading books
   c. Watching cartoons
   d. Role playing

Part V – Insurance, Records and Bookkeeping

1. What type of Medical Insurance plan does the employer typically pay?

   a. Health Maintenance Organization (HMO)
   b. Indemnity
   c. Major Medical
   d. None of the Above

2. Preferred Provider Organization (PPO) insurance:

   a. is a list of health care providers that provided services at a discounted rate.
   b. does not cover primary care.
   c. usually has deductibles and limits.
   d. does not offer a discounted rate.

3. Which program offers health care to dependents and spouses of service women and men?

    a. Medigap
    b. Tricare
    c. Commercial Insurance
    d. CHAMPVA

4. What Medical plan is for people over 65?

    a. Medicaid
    b. Tricare
    c. CHAMPVA
    d. Medicare

5. What is an RVU?

    a. the system for reimbursement.
    b. a component that is multiplied by a monetary conversion factor to calculate physicians costs.
    c. a list of procedures.
    d. a list of procedures and their cost.

6. What is the insured person's child called?

    a. coinsured
    b. dependent
    c. group insured member
    d. family insured member

7. What is the 'point of service?'

   a. The place where they bought the insurance.

   b. The place where the patient was injured.

   c. The place where the service is delivered.

   d. The place where they pay for the service.

8. What is precertification?

   a. getting approval for a service or procedure

   b. determining if the service is covered

   c. determining the amount the insurance company will cover

   d. None of the Above

9. What type of insurance covers significant illness?

   a. Medicare

   b. Major Medical

   c. Indemnity

   d. HMO

10. Medicare Part A covers

   a. hospital inpatient costs

   b. hospital outpatient costs

   c. No hospital costs

   d. Doctor office visits

11. Medicare Part B covers

   a. physician costs

   b. outpatient services

   c. physician costs

   d. physician costs

12. Which of the following are NOT eligible for TRICARE:

a. Veterans
b. Army service men and women
c. Special Forces men and women
d. Spouses of service men or women convicted of spousal or child abuse

13. Which of the following is NOT a benefit under Worker's Compensation?

a. Prostheses
b. Spousal treatment
c. Death Benefits to Survivors
d. Permanent disability payments

14. Which of the following methods of insurance payment is based on a relative value system?

a. Fee Schedule
b. RBRVS
c. UCR
d. Capitation

15. What is included on the Day Sheet?

a. Charges and payments received
b. Patients and doctors names
c. Itemized statement of a patient's accounts receivable
d. List of all monies owed

16. What type of account is the Day Sheet?

a. Accounts Payable
b. General Ledger
c. Accounts Receivable
d. Patient Ledger

17. A medical office has run out of pencils and paper. How should you purchase these?

    a. With a company check.

    b. With petty cash.

    c. With your own funds and ask for reimbursement.

    d. With cash from the cash box.

18. All funds owed for items such as rent are:

    a. Accounts Receivable

    b. Accounts Payable

    c. Receipts

    d. General Ledger items

19. What form would a courier issue to the office upon receipt of a package?

    a. Invoice

    b. Receipt

    c. Bill of Lading

    d. Purchase Order

20. Funds owed to a physician from patients and others are called

    a. Account Receivable

    b. Account Payable

    c. Net Income

    d. Expenses

21. What form has all the information for a patient to file an insurance claim?

    a. Superbill
    b. Invoice
    c. Receipt
    d. Ledger

22. A Debit to an account:

    a. is an amount owed.
    b. is an amount paid.
    c. None of the above.

23. The amount of income a physician's office makes after taxes and expenses is:

    a. Gross Income
    b. Wage
    c. Gross expenses
    d. Net income

24. Comparing the checkbook to the bank statement is called

    a. Auditing
    b. Reconciliation
    c. Balancing
    d. Account balancing

Part VI – Fundamental Writing Skills

1. Choose the sentence below with the correct punctuation.

    a. To make chicken soup you must first buy a chicken.

    b. To make chicken soup you must first, buy a chicken.

    c. To make chicken soup, you must first buy a chicken.

    d. To make chicken soup; you must first buy a chicken.

2. Choose the sentence below with the correct punctuation.

    a. To travel around the globe you have to drive 25,000 miles.

    b. To travel around the globe, you have to drive 25000 miles.

    c. To travel around the globe, you have to drive, 25000 miles.

    d. To travel around the globe, you have to drive 25,000 miles.

3. Choose the sentence below with the correct punctuation.

    a. The dog loved chasing bones, but never ate them; it was running that he enjoyed.

    b. The dog loved chasing bones; but never ate them, it was running that he enjoyed.

    c. The dog loved chasing bones, but never ate them, it was running that he enjoyed.

    d. The dog loved chasing bones; but never ate them: it was running that he enjoyed.

4. Choose the sentence below with the correct punctuation.

a. He had not paid the rent, therefore, the landlord changed the locks.

b. He had not paid the rent; therefore, the landlord changed the locks.

c. He had not paid the rent, therefore; the landlord changed the locks.

d. He had not paid the rent therefore, the landlord changed the locks.

5. Choose the sentence with the correct grammar.

a. He would have postponed the camping trip, if he would have known about the forecast.

b. If he would have known about the forecast, he would have postponed the camping trip.

c. If he have known about the forecast, he would have postponed the camping trip.

d. If he had known about the forecast, he would have postponed the camping trip.

6. Choose the sentence with the correct grammar.

a. If Joe had told me the truth, I wouldn't have been so angry.

b. If Joe would have told me the truth, I wouldn't have been so angry.

c. I wouldn't have been so angry if Joe would have told the truth.

d. If Joe would have telled me the truth, I wouldn't have been so angry.

7. Choose the sentence with the correct grammar.

a. He doesn't have any money to buy clothes and neither do I.

b. He doesn't have any money to buy clothes and neither does I.

c. He don't have any money to buy clothes and neither do I.

d. He don't have any money to buy clothes and neither does I.

8. Choose the sentence with the correct grammar.

a. Because it really don't matter, I don't care if I go there.

b. Because it really doesn't matter, I doesn't care if I go there.

c. Because it really doesn't matter, I don't care if I go there.

d. Because it really don't matter, I don't care if I go there.

9. Choose the sentence with the correct grammar.

a. When we go to the picnic, we will take potato salad and wieners.

b. If you come to the picnic, bring potato salad and wieners.

c. When we go to the picnic, we will bring potato salad and wieners.

d. If you come to the picnic, take potato salad and wieners.

10. Choose the sentence with the correct grammar.

a. Until you take the overdue books to the library, you can't take any new ones home

b. Until you take the overdue books to the library, you can't bring any new ones home.

c. Until you bring the overdue books to the library, you can't take any new ones home.

d. Until you take the overdue books to the library, you can't take any new ones home.

11. Choose the sentence with the correct grammar.

a. Newer cars use fewer gasoline, and produce fewer emissions.

b. Newer cars use less gasoline, and produce less emissions.

c. Newer cars use less gasoline, and produce fewer emissions.

d. Newer cars fewer less gasoline, and produce less emissions.

12. Choose the sentence with the correct grammar.

a. His doctor suggested that he eat less snacks and do fewer lounging on the couch.

b. His doctor suggested that he eat fewer snacks and do less lounging on the couch.

c. His doctor suggested that he eat less snacks and do less lounging on the couch.

d. His doctor suggested that he eat fewer snacks and do fewer lounging on the couch.

13. Choose the sentence with the correct grammar.

a. However, I believe that he didn't really try that hard.
b. However I believe that he didn't really try that hard.
c. However; I believe that he didn't really try that hard.
d. However: I believe that he didn't really try that hard.

14. Choose the sentence with the correct grammar.

a. There was however, very little difference between the two.

b. There was, however very little difference between the two.

c. There was; however, very little difference between the two.

d. There was, however, very little difference between the two.

15. Choose the sentence with the correct grammar.

a. Don would never have thought of that book, but you could have reminded him.

b. Don would never of thought of that book, but you could have reminded him.

c. Don would never have thought of that book, but you could of have reminded him.

d. Don would never of thought of that book, but you could of reminded him.

16. Choose the sentence with the correct grammar.

a. The mother would not of punished her daughter if she could have avoided it.

b. The mother would not have punished her daughter if she could of avoided it.

c. The mother would not of punished her daughter if she could of avoided it.

d. The mother would not have punished her daughter if she could have avoided it.

17. Choose the sentence with the correct usage.

a. Even with an speed limit sign clearly posted, an inattentive driver may drive too fast.

b. Even with a speed limit sign clearly posted, a inattentive driver may drive too fast.

c. Even with an speed limit sign clearly posted, a inattentive driver may drive too fast.

d. Even with a speed limit sign clearly posted, an inattentive driver may drive too fast.

18. Choose the sentence with the correct usage.

a. Except for the roses, she did not accept John's frequent gifts.

b. Accept for the roses, she did not except John's frequent gifts.

c. Accept for the roses, she did not accept John's frequent gifts.

d. Except for the roses, she did not except John's frequent gifts.

19. Choose the sentence with the correct usage.

a. Although he continued to advise me, I no longer took his advice.

b. Although he continued to advice me, I no longer took his advise.

c. Although he continued to advise me, I no longer took his advise.

d. Although he continued to advice me, I no longer took his advise.

20. Choose the sentence with the correct usage.

a. In order to adopt to the climate, we had to adopt a different style of clothing.

b. In order to adapt to the climate, we had to adapt a different style of clothing.

c. In order to adapt to the climate, we had to adopt a different style of clothing.

d. In order to adapt to the climate, we had to adapt a different style of clothing.

21. Choose the sentence with the correct usage.

a. When he's between friends, Robert seems confident, but, between you and me, he is really very shy.

b. When he's among friends, Robert seems confident, but, among you and me, he is really very shy.

c. When he's between friends, Robert seems confident, but, among you and me, he is really very shy.

d. When he's among friends, Robert seems confident, but, between you and me, he is really very shy.

22. Choose the sentence with the correct usage.

a. I will be finished at ten in the morning, and will be arriving at home at about 6:30.

b. I will be finished at about ten in the morning, and will be arriving at home at 6:30.

c. I will be finished at about ten in the morning, and will be arriving at home at about 6:30.

d. I will be finished at ten in the morning, and will be arriving at home at 6:30.

23. Choose the sentence with the correct usage.

a. Beside the red curtains and pillows, there was a red rug beside the couch.

b. Besides the red curtains and pillows, there was a red rug beside the couch.

c. Besides the red curtains and pillows, there was a red rug besides the couch.

d. Beside the red curtains and pillows, there was a red rug besides the couch.

24. Choose the sentence with the correct usage.

a. Although John can swim very well, the lifeguard may not allow him to swim in the pool.

b. Although John may swim very well, the lifeguard may not allow him to swim in the pool.

c. Although John can swim very well, the lifeguard can not allow him to swim in the pool.

d. Although John may swim very well, the lifeguard may not allow him to swim in the pool.

25. Choose the sentence with the correct usage.

a. Her continuous absences caused a continual disruption at the office.

b. Her continual absences caused a continuous disruption at the office.

c. Her continual absences caused a continual disruption at the office.

d. Her continuous absences caused a continuous disruption at the office.

26. Choose the sentence with the correct usage.

a. During the famine, the Irish people had to emigrate to other countries; many of them immigrated to the United States.

b. During the famine, the Irish people had to immigrate to other countries; many of them immigrated to the United States.

c. During the famine, the Irish people had to emigrate to other countries; many of them emigrated to the United States.

d. During the famine, the Irish people had to immigrate to other countries; many of them emigrated to the United States.

27. Choose the sentence with the correct usage.

a. His home was farther than we expected; farther, the roads were very bad.

b. His home was farther than we expected; further, the roads were very bad.

c. His home was further than we expected; further, the roads were very bad.

d. His home was further than we expected; farther, the roads were very bad.

28. **Choose the sentence with the correct usage.**

   a. The volunteers brought groceries and toys to the homeless shelter; the latter were given to the staff, while the former were given directly to the children.

   b. The volunteers brought groceries and toys to the homeless shelter; the former was given to the staff, while the latter was given directly to the children.

   c. The volunteers brought groceries and toys to the homeless shelter; the groceries were given to the staff, while the former was given directly to the children.

   d. The volunteers brought groceries and toys to the homeless shelter; the latter was given to the staff, while the groceries were given directly to the children.

29. **Choose the sentence with the correct usage.**

   a. You shouldn't sit in that chair wearing black pants; I set the white cat there just a moment ago.

   b. You shouldn't set in that chair wearing black pants; I sit the white cat there just a moment ago.

   c. You shouldn't set in that chair wearing black pants; I set the white cat there just a moment ago.

   d. You shouldn't sit in that chair wearing black pants; I sit the white cat there just a moment ago.

30. **Choose the sentence with the correct capitalization.**

   a. Mars is the god or war.

   b. Mars is the God of war.

   c. Mars is the God of War.

   d. Mars is the god of war.

31. Choose the sentence with the correct capitalization.

a. This is her third term as mayor of Chicago.
b. This is her third term as Mayor of Chicago.
c. This is her third term as mayor of chicago.
d. None of the above.

32. Choose the sentence with the correct capitalization.

a. I was able to speak with Susan Roberts, Mayor of Tampa.
b. I was able to speak with Susan Roberts, mayor of Tampa.
c. I was able to speak with Susan Roberts, Mayor of tampa.
d. None of the Above.

33. Choose the sentence with the correct capitalization.

a. I think thanksgiving is the best fall holiday.
b. I think Thanksgiving is the best Fall holiday.
c. I think Thanksgiving is the best fall holiday.
d. None of the above.

34. Choose the sentence with the correct capitalization.

a. I will be skipping the Fall 2012 Semester.
b. I will be skipping the fall 2012 semester.
c. I will be skipping the Fall 2012 semester.
d. None of the above.

35. Choose the sentence with the correct capitalization.

    a. They speak Spanish in Mexico.
    b. They speak spanish in Mexico.
    c. They speak spanish in mexico.
    d. None of the above.

Answer Key

Part I – Medical Terminology

1. D
Enemas are never administered to prepare patients for surgery.

2. A
A **radical prostatectomy** is a procedure in which both the **prostate gland** and some of the surrounding tissue are excised to eliminate cancer or to treat **benign prostatic hyperplasia** or an **enlarged prostate**.

3. D
The **gall bladder** is a pear-shaped sac located near the right lobe of the liver that holds **bile**; a/an **cholecystectomy** is surgery to remove that organ.

4. A
In cases of bladder stones or the removal of other tissue from the bladder, a/an **Cystoscopy** is performed by the insertion of a thin, lighted instrument through the urethra and into the bladder.

5. D
An **Arthroscopy** allows a physician to examine the surfaces of the joints and surrounding tissues to diagnose joint complications, repair injuries, remove foreign bodies or monitor disease.

6. C
Decompressive laminectomy is the most frequently performed surgery for the treatment of spinal stenosis; the procedure relieves pressure on the spinal cord caused by age-related changes in the spine.

7. D
Alternatives for the treatment of breast cancer include either **simple** or **modified radical lumpectomy** or a **mastectomy** followed by radiation treatment.

8. D
Bodily organs can sometimes adhere to the **peritoneum**, a two-layered membrane lining the abdominal cavity and covering abdominal organs; when this occurs, it the problem is corrected through surgical release of **peritoneal** adhesions.

9. A
A standard liver panel are a group of tests that are performed together to detect, evaluate, and monitor disease or damage. This procedure determines levels of albumin and bilirubin, among others.

10. D
A/an **Enzyme Linked Immunosorbent Assay (ELISA.** refers to the test usually used to screen for HIV infection.

11. C
The following statement is false: **Ultrasound imaging is less effective than x-rays at revealing soft tissue damage such as torn ligaments, muscles and tendons.**

12. B
A/an **complete blood count (CBC.** provides information about the number and percentage of red and white blood cells and platelets present. Because abnormally high or low counts indicate many types of disease, this test is one of the most commonly performed blood tests in medicine.

13. A
Testing for genetic defects is possible using **amniocentesis,** usually done at 14 to 16 weeks of pregnancy.

14. D
All the statements are true.

15. B
Radiography diagnostic procedure used equipment to develop an image clearly displaying areas of differing density and composition.

16. C
A **blood culture** is a microbiological culture of blood used to

detect infections such as bacteria and septicemia.

17. Endocrinology is a branch of medicine that deals with the **endocrine** system and its production of hormones, which coordinate metabolism, respiration, and excretion, among others. Medical professionals in this field treat persons with diabetes, thyroid diseases, cholesterol disorders, and metabolic disorders.

18. C
A geriatrician's practice is limited to persons over the age of 65 is false. Geriatrics is a sub-specialty of internal medicine and family medicine that focuses on health care of elderly people. It aims to promote health by preventing and treating diseases and disabilities in older adults. There is no set age at which patients may be under the care of a geriatrician, or physician who specializes in the care of elderly people. Rather, this decision is determined by the individual patient's needs, and the availability of a specialist.[1]

19. A
Hepatology is the medical specialty involved in the study of the liver, gallbladder, biliary tree, and pancreas and diseases such as viral hepatitis and alcohol-related conditions.

20. D
Oral and Maxillofacial surgeons use their skills to correct diseases, defects and injuries in the head, neck, face, jaws and the hard and soft tissues of the oral and facial region.

21. A
Palliative medicine is another name for hospice care is false.

Palliative care is a specialized area of healthcare that focuses on relieving and preventing the suffering of patients. Unlike hospice care, palliative medicine is appropriate for patients in all disease stages, including those undergoing treatment for curable illnesses and those living with chronic diseases, as well as patients who are nearing the end of life. Palliative medicine utilizes a multidisciplinary approach to patient care, relying on input from physicians, pharmacists, nurses, chaplains, social workers, psychologists, and other allied health professionals in formulating a plan of care to relieve suffering in all areas of a patient's life.[2]

22. C
Nephrology concerns the diagnosis and treatment of kidney diseases, including electrolyte disturbances and hypertension, and the care of those requiring renal replacement therapy, including dialysis and renal transplant patients.[3]

23. C
Oncology is a branch of medicine that deals with cancer. A medical professional who practices oncology is an oncologist. Oncology is concerned with:

- The diagnosis of any cancer in a person
- Therapy (e.g., surgery, chemotherapy, radiotherapy and other modalities)
- Follow-up of cancer patients after successful treatment
- Palliative care of patients with terminal malignancies
- Ethical questions surrounding cancer care

Screening efforts:
of populations, or of the relatives of patients (in types of cancer that are thought to have a hereditary basis, such as breast cancer)[4]

24. B
Pathology is the precise study and diagnosis of disease.

Pathology addresses 4 components of disease: cause/etiology, mechanisms of development (pathogenesis), structural alterations of cells (morphologic changes), and the consequences of changes (clinical manifestations).
Pathology is further separated into divisions, based on either the system being studied (e.g. veterinary pathology and animal disease) or the focus of the examination (e.g. forensic pathology and determining the cause of death).[5]

25. B
The greek root -pepsia means digestion. For example, dyspepsia.

26. A
The Greek root -apathy means disease. Examples include homeopathy and naprapathy.

27. B
The Latin root abdomin- means the abdomen area. An example is abdominal.

28. C
The Greek and Latin root aort means aorta.

29. A
The Greek root brachi means arm. For example, brachium (i.e., the upper arm).

30. C
The Greek root arteri means artery. For xample, arteriosclerosis and arteries.

31. B
The Latin root dors- means back. For example, dorsal and dorsum.

32. C
The Latin root allic- means big toe.

33. A
The Greek root cyst(o)- means bladder. For example, Cystectomy, a procedure to remove the bladder.

34. C
The Greek root hemat- means blooFor example, Hemophilia, a blood-coagulation disorder.

35. A
The Greek root thromb(o)- means blood clot. For example, thrombosis, the formation of a blood clot.

36. D
The Greek root angio- means blood vessels. For example, Angioplasty, a procedure in which blood vessels are widened.

37. B
The Greek root stetho- means chest. For example, stethoscope, an instrument that is often used to listen to the heart by placing the end of it on the chest.

38. C
The Latin root aur- means relating to the ear. For example, the auditory canal is a part of the inner ear.

39. B
The Greek root ophthalmo- means relating to the eyes. For example, an ophthalmologist is an eye doctor.

40. A
The Greek root lipo- means relating to fat. For example, liposuction is a procedure in which fat is surgically removed.

41. C
The Latin root digit- means relating to fingers. Our use of the word "digits" to signifiy numbers comes from the practice of counting on one's fingers - or digits.

42. B
The Latin root manu- means relating to the hanFor example, "manuscript" refers to a written text that was printed by hand.

43. A
The Greek root cardi- means relating to the heart. For example, cardiac arrest is a heart attack.

44. B
The Greek root entero- means relating to the intestine. For example, enteroclysis is an X-ray of the patient's small intestine.

45. C
The Latin root ren- means relating to the kidney. For example, renal failure is kidney failure.

46. A
The Greek root trachel means relating to the neck. For example, the trachea is located in the throat.

47. C
The Greek root neuro- means relating to the nerves. For example, a neurologist is a doctor who specializes in diagnosis and treatment of nerve disorders.

48. B
The Greek root medi- in anatomy or other areas, means the middle.
Examples include medium and median.

49. A
The Latin root equi in anatomy or other areas, means equal. For example, equilibrium, equidistant and equivalent.

50. B
The Latin prefix ab-, in a medical context, means away from. For example, absorb, to suck away.

51. C
The Greek prefix aesthesio-, in a medical context, means sensation. For example, anesthesia (it replaces the sensation of pain with a more pleasurable one) and aesthetic (value based on how it pleases the senses).

52. A
The Greek prefix bio-, in a medical context, means life. For example, biology, biography and biochemical (chemicals developed from life forms).

53. D
The Latin prefix capit- means head. For example, decapitate (to remove someone's head. and capital (the main city or "head" of a state).

54. A
The Latin prefix carp-, in a medical context, means wrist. For example, Carpal Tunnel Syndrome (nerve pain felt primarily in the wrists) and carpopedal (a problem that affects the wrist and the foot).

55. B
The Greek prefix cata-, in a medical context, means down or under. For example, cataracts, also, catacombs (passages under the ground..

56. C
The Latin prefix dis-, in a medical context, means taking something apart or separating. For example, dissect (to cut a body apart) and disembody (separating one's mind or spirit from his body).

57. B
The Greek prefix endo-, in a medical context, means inside or within. For example, endospore and endocrinology.

58. A
The Greek prefix exo-, in a medical context, means outside. For example, exoskeleton (a skeleton on the outside of the body) and exobiotic (living on the outside of a substrate or on the outside of a living organism.

59. C
The prefix fibro-, in a medical context, means fiber. For example, fibroblast and fibromyalgia.

60. A
The prefix filli-, in a medical context, means hair-like or fine. For example, filament.

Part II – Anatomy and Physiology

1. C
The abdomen can be divided by two lines into 4 quadrants or by 4 lines into 9 regions.

The two lines that divide the abdomen into quadrants form a cross, the centre of which is positioned over the umbilicus (belly button). These quadrants are often used to indicate the location of pain.

Quadrant Name	Contains
Right upper quadrant	Liver, gallbladder, right kidney, duodenum, a portion of the ascending and transverse colons and the small intestine.

Left upper quadrant	Stomach, spleen, left kidney, pancreas, a portion of the descending and transverse colons and the small intestine.
Right lower quadrant	Appendix, caecum, a potion of the ascending colon and the small intestine.
Left lower quadrant	A portion of the descending and transverse colons and the small intestine.

2. A
The Left upper quadrant of the abdomen, is often abbreviated as LUQ, contains the stomach, spleen, left lobe of the liver, body of the pancreas, left kidney and adrenal gland.

3. D
The right upper quadrant of the abdomen, often abbreviated as RUQ, contains the liver, gall bladder, duodenum and had of the pancreas.

4. A
The Right lower quadrant of the human abdomen, often abbreviated as RLQ, contains the appendix and ascending colon.

5. B
Medical personnel divide the abdomen into smaller regions to facilitate study and discussion.

6. A
The stomach and colon are both in the Left Upper Quadrant, together with, liver, spleen, left kidney, pancreas and large intestine.

7. C
The commonly used abbreviations for the Quadrants are, Right Upper Quadrant, RUQ, Left Upper Quadrant, LUQ, Right Lower Quadrant, RLQ, Left Lower Quadrant, LLQ.

8. D
All of the above. The Large Intestine passes through all the

quadrants.

9. B
The stomach and colon are both in the Left Upper Quadrant, together with, liver, spleen, left kidney, pancreas and large intestine.

10. A
The gallbladder is located in the Right Upper Quadrant together with the liver, right kidney, colon, pancreas and large intestine.

11. D
The human body manages a multitude of highly complex interactions to maintain balance within a normal range. The kidneys are responsible for regulating blood water levels, re-absorption of substances into the blood, maintenance of salt and ion levels in the blood, regulation of blood pH, and excretion of urea and other wastes.[6]

12. A
Homeostasis is the property of a system that regulates its internal environment and tends to maintain a stable, constant condition of properties like temperature or pH.

13. D
The amount of energy / calories that your body requires to maintain itself is **metabolism.**

14. B
Exercise and low fat diets will increase metabolism. Choice B, **a man who is past 30 and whose body is losing muscle** is the only choice.

15. A
Exercise will increase metabolism, so **aerobic exercise**.

16. A
The kidneys are responsible for regulating fluid balance.

17. B
Fluid balance is important, because **water** comprises about 60-70% of a person's weight.

18. B
Metabolism slows with aging.

19. D
"Met" refers to **the person's metabolic rate.**

20. A
Fluid balance is important, because the human body loses water every day through urination, perspiration, feces, and **breathing**.

21. D
The smallest unit of life in our bodies is the **cell**.

22. B
The cell membrane or plasma membrane is a biological membrane that separates the interior of all cells from the outside environment. The cell membrane is selectively permeable to ions and organic molecules and controls the movement of substances in and out of cells.[7]

23. A
Cell division is the process by which a parent cell divides into two or more daughter cells. Cell division is usually a small segment of a larger cell cycle.

24. C
Mitosis is the process by which a eukaryotic cell separates the chromosomes in its cell nucleus into two identical sets in two separate nuclei. The process of mitosis is fast and highly complex. The sequence of events is divided into stages corresponding to the completion of one set of activities and the start of the next. These stages are interphase, prophase, prometaphase, metaphase, anaphase and telophase.[8]

25. B
Mitosis is the process by which a eukaryotic cell separates the chromosomes in its cell nucleus into two identical sets in two separate nuclei.[8]

26. A
Prophase, is a stage of mitosis in which the chromatin condenses (it becomes shorter and fatter) into a highly

ordered structure called a chromosome in which the chromatin becomes visible.[9]

27. B
Metaphase is a stage of mitosis in the eukaryotic cell cycle in which condensed & highly coiled chromosomes, carrying genetic information, align in the middle of the cell before being separated into each of the two daughter cells. Preceded by events in prometaphase and followed by anaphase, microtubules formed in prophase have already found and attached themselves to kinetochores in metaphase.[10]

28. D
Anaphase is the stage of mitosis or meiosis when chromosomes move to opposite poles of the cell. Anaphase begins with the regulated triggering of the metaphase-to-anaphase transition. Metaphase ends with the destruction of cyclin, which is required for the function of metaphase cyclin-dependent kinases (M-Cdks). Anaphase is initiated with the cleavage of securin, a protein that inhibits the protease known as separase. Separase then cleaves cohesin, a protein responsible for holding sister chromatids together.[11]

29. D
Telophase is a stage in both meiosis and mitosis in an eukaryotic cell. During telophase, the effects of prophase and prometaphase events are reversed. Two daughter nuclei form in the cell. The nuclear envelopes of the daughter cells are formed from the fragments of the nuclear envelope of the parent cell. As the nuclear envelope forms around each pair of chromatids, the nucleoli reappear.[12]

30. B
Epithelium is one of the four basic types of animal tissue, along with connective tissue, muscle tissue and nervous tissue. Epithelial tissues line the cavities and surfaces of structures throughout the body, and form many glands. Functions of epithelial cells include secretion, selective absorption, protection, transcellular transport and detection of sensation.

The shape of their cells generally classifies simple epithelial tissues. The four major classes of simple epithelium are: (1) simple squamous; (2) simple cuboidal; (3) simple columnar; (4) pseudostratified.[13]

31. B
Epithelial tissue **acts as a protective barrier for the human body.**

32. C
The functions of connective tissue are, storage of energy, protection of organs, providing structural framework for the body and connection of body tissues.

33. C
Muscle tissue can **relax and contract**, bringing out movement and the ability to work.

34. D
Nervous tissue is specialized to **react to stimuli**.

35. A
Nerve tissue is made of cells called neurons.

36. C
The integumentary system is the organ system that protects the body from damage, comprising the skin and its appendages, including hair, scales, feathers, and nails.

37. C
The integumentary system comprises the **skin** and its various appendages, including hair, scales, feathers, and nails.

38. B
The appendages of the integumentary system are hair, scales, feathers, and nails.

39. D
The integumentary system has a variety of functions; it may serve to waterproof, cushion, and protect the deeper tissues, excrete wastes, and **regulate temperature**, and is the attachment site for sensory receptors to detect pain, sensation, pressure, and temperature.

40. C
The human skin (integumentary) is composed of a minimum of 3 major layers of tissue, the Epidermis, the Dermis and Hypodermis.[14]

41. D
The human skin (integumentary) is composed of a minimum of 3 major layers of tissue, the Epidermis, the Dermis and Hypodermis.[14]

42. A
The **dermis** is the middle layer of skin, composed of dense irregular connective tissues such as collagen with elastin arranged in a diffusely bundled and woven pattern. These layers give elasticity to the integument, allowing stretching and conferring flexibility, while also resisting distortions, wrinkling, and sagging.[14]

43. B
Acne is an example of a minor ailment of the integumentary system.

44. B
Skin cancer is an example of a serious ailment of the integumentary system.

45. C.
Musculoskeletal is a body system comprised mostly of the bones.

46. B.
Joints are an example of **connective tissue** within the musculoskeletal system.

47. A
One of the primary purposes of the musculoskeletal system is **providing stability to the body**.

48. D
Another primary purpose of the musculoskeletal system is **providing form for the body**.

49. C
It is difficult to diagnose an ailment within the musculoskeletal system because of its close proximity to other organs.

50. A
Cartilage is a flexible connective tissue found in many areas in the bodies of humans and other animals, including the joints between bones, the rib cage, the ear, the nose, the elbow, the knee, the ankle, the bronchial tubes and the intervertebral discs. It is not as hard and rigid as bone but is stiffer and less flexible than muscle.[15]

Part III – Medical Law, Ethics and Legislation

1. D
Medical ethics is a system of moral principles that apply values and judgments to the practice of medicine. As a scholarly discipline, medical ethics encompasses its practical application in clinical settings as well as work on its history, philosophy, theology, and sociology.

2. D
All the statements are true.

> The patient has been given false information about a treatment.
> The patient is judged incompetent to consent to treatment and has received improper care.
> Care that the patient has refused is forced on them without court authorization.

Battery is a criminal offense involving unlawful physical contact, distinct from assault, which is the fear of such contact.

In the United States, criminal battery, or simply battery, is the use of force against another, resulting in harmful or offensive contact. It is a specific common law misdemeanor, although the term is used more generally to refer to any unlawful offensive physical contact with another person, and may be a misdemeanor or a felony, depending on the circumstances. Battery is "any unlawful touching of the person of another by the aggressor himself, or by a substance put in motion by him." Often, battery is now governed by statute, and its severity is determined by the law of the specific jurisdiction.[17]

3. A
The four major principles of medical ethics are **autonomy, beneficence, non-malfeasance and justice.**

Autonomy - the patient has the right to refuse or choose their treatment.
Beneficence - a practitioner should act in the best interest of the patient.
Non-malfeasance - "first, do no harm."
Justice - concerns the distribution of scarce health resources, and the decision of who gets what treatment (fairness and equality).

Values such as these do not give answers as to how to handle a particular situation, but provide a useful framework for understanding conflicts.[17]

4. B
Double effect does NOT state that, the action being considered is in itself either morally good or morally indifferent.

The principle of double effect; also known as the rule of double effect; the doctrine of double effect, often abbreviated as DDE or PDE; double-effect reasoning; or simply double effect, is a set of ethical criteria for evaluating the permissibility of acting when one's otherwise legitimate act (for example, relieving a terminally ill patient's pain) will also cause an effect one would normally be obliged to avoid (for example, the patient's death).

This set of criteria states that an action having foreseen harmful effects practically inseparable from the good effect is justifiable if upon satisfaction of the following:

- the nature of the act is itself good, or at least morally neutral;
- the agent intends the good effect and not the bad either as a means to the good or as an end itself;
- the good effect outweighs the bad effect in circumstances sufficiently grave to justify causing the bad effect and the agent exercises due diligence to minimize the harm. (Double-Effect Reasoning: Doing Good and Avoiding Evil, p.36, Oxford: Clarendon Press, T. A. Cavanaugh)[19]

5. D
The following statements about the AMT standards of practice are false:

- Only duly licensed physicians/dentists are required to report any knowledge of professional abuse to the appropriate authorities.
- The judgment of the attending physician/dentist shall be protected and valued, no matter what the circumstances.

6. D
Confidentiality is an ethical principle that states that communication between a patient and a provider must remain private.

7. D
Beneficence is the major principle of medical ethics that states that physicians and other medical professionals must act in the best interest of the patient.

The term beneficence refers to actions that promote the well being of others. In the medical context, this means taking actions that serve the best interests of patients. However, uncertainty surrounds the precise definition of which practices do in fact help patients.[20]

8. A
The principles of **autonomy** and **privacy** must be balanced

to be certain that any risks involved in medical treatment or procedures is outweighed by the benefit to the patient.

9. A
Justice concerns the distribution of scarce health resources, and the decision of who gets what treatment (fairness and equality).

10. D
A **triage** system is a process by which treatment is prioritized based on needed personnel and those who are most critically ill or injured.

Triage is the process of determining the priority of patients' treatments based on the severity of their condition. This rations patient treatment efficiently when resources are insufficient for all to be treated immediately. Two types of triage exist: simple and advanced. Triage may result in determining the order and priority of emergency treatment, the order and priority of emergency transport, or the transport destination for the patient.
Triage may also be used for patients arriving at the emergency department, or to telephone medical advice systems, among others.[21]

11. D
Informed consent is a phrase often used in law to indicate that the consent a person gives meets certain minimum standards. As a literal matter, in the absence of fraud, it is redundant. An informed consent can be said to have been given based upon a clear appreciation and understanding of the facts, implications, and future consequences of an action. In order to give informed consent, the individual concerned must have adequate reasoning faculties and be in possession of all relevant facts at the time consent is given. Impairments to reasoning and judgment which may make it impossible for someone to give informed consent include such factors as basic intellectual or emotional immaturity, high levels of stress such as PTSD or as severe mental retardation, severe mental illness, intoxication, severe sleep deprivation, Alzheimer's disease, or being in a coma.[22]

12. A
Before a common procedure with little risk such as a blood test or in an emergency, life-threatening situation are exceptions to the rule of informed consent.

13. D
Before a patient exercises their right to refusal of treatment, they must be informed about:

- The diagnosis and prognosis of their medical condition
- Available alternative treatments and the risks and benefits of those options
- The risk and probable outcome of no intervention

14. A
Legally mandated treatment is medical care or testing without their permission.

15. D
The situations in which patients must submit to legally mandated treatments include:

- The patient has been judged incompetent and has been appointed a guardian.
- The patient has been involuntarily confined to a mental institution.
- A court has ordered treatment under the authority of public health laws.

16. B
A **therapeutic exception** is an exception to the requirement of informed consent and allows the withholding of information from a patient if such information would cause psychological damage and therefore endanger their physical well-being.

17. B
The following statement about medical malpractice is false, a medical malpractice suit can be filed any time that patient consent was not obtained before treatment.

Medical malpractice is professional negligence by act or

omission by a health care provider in which the treatment provided falls below the accepted standard of practice in the medical community and causes injury or death to the patient, with most cases involving medical error. Standards and regulations for medical malpractice vary by country and jurisdiction within countries. Medical professionals may obtain professional liability insurances to offset the risk and costs of lawsuits based on medical malpractice.[23]

18. C
Torts result in criminal trials that assess guilt or innocence is false.

A tort, in common law jurisdictions, is a wrong that involves a breach of a civil duty (other than a contractual duty) owed to someone else. It is differentiated from a crime, which involves a breach of a duty owed to society in general. Though many acts are both torts and crimes, the State usually prosecutes crimes, whereas a person who has been injured may bring a lawsuit or tort. [24]

19. C
An **advance directive** is a legal document filed in advance by a patient which details their wishes if they are incapacitated.

An advance health care directive, also known as living will, personal directive, advance directive, or advance decision, are instructions given by individuals specifying what actions they wish taken in the event they are no longer able to make decisions due to illness or incapacity, and appoints a person to make such decisions on their behalf. A living will is one form of advance directive, leaving instructions for treatment. Another form authorizes a specific type of power of attorney or health care proxy, where the individual appoints someone to make decisions on their behalf when they are incapacitated. People may also have a combination of both. It is often encouraged that people complete both documents to provide the most comprehensive guidance regarding their care. One example of a combination document is the Five Wishes advance directive in the United States.[25]

20. D
The following are true about living wills:

- They are documents in which the patient chooses a surrogate who can make healthcare decisions if they are incapacitated.
- They demand that no extraordinary measures such as CPR, are used in an effort to revive the patient.

21. D
Two types of advance directives are **a living will and a durable power of attorney.**

An advance health care directive, also known as living will, personal directive, advance directive, or advance decision, are instructions given by individuals specifying what actions they wish taken in the event that they are no longer able to make decisions due to illness or incapacity, and appoints a person to make such decisions on their behalf. A living will is one form of advance directive, leaving instructions for treatment. Another form authorizes a specific type of power of attorney or health care proxy, where someone is appointed by the individual to make decisions on their behalf when they are incapacitated. People may also have a combination of both. It is often encouraged that people complete both documents to provide the most comprehensive guidance regarding their care. One example of a combination document is the Five Wishes advance directive in the United States.[25]

22. A
Besides state laws, the Uniform Anatomical Gift Act is the law that governs the donation of organs and tissues.

The Uniform Anatomical Gift Act governs organ donations for the purpose of transplantation, and governs anatomical gifts of one's own cadaver for dissection and study. The law provides that in the absence of such a document, a surviving spouse, or if there is no spouse, a list of specific relatives in order of preference, can make the gift. It also seeks to limit the liability of health care providers who act on good faith representations that a deceased patient meant to make an anatomical gift. The act also prohibits trafficking and trafficking in human organs for profit from donations for transplant or therapy.[26]

23. B
While **negligence** is a mistake or a failure to be careful, **malpractice** includes wrongful conduct by a professional or a failure to meet standards of care that results in harm to another person.

24. D
All these conditions prevent organ or tissue donation:

   Advanced age and metastatic cancer
   A history of hepatitis, HIV or AIDS
   Sepsis

25. C
In **whole brain death**, the brain no longer functions organically and the patient is kept alive by artificial means. When a patient's cerebrum is dead and they are unconscious, cannot think or reason, but May still be breathing, they have experienced **higher brain death**.

26. C
OSHA stands for Occupational Safety and Health Administration. OSHA is an agency within the U.S. Department of Labor created as part of the Occupational Safety and Health Act.

27. A
OSHA's chief function is overseeing private sector workplaces to prevent possible dangers or hazards that could affect workers.

28. C
An example of OSHA initiating an inspection is when workers have complained about a hazard in the worksite. A large percentage of OSHA inspections originate when the workers file a complaint.

29. A
OSHA demands that all employers comply with their final rules published under the 1970 Occupational Safety and Health Act.

30. A
FDA stands for Food and Drug Administration. It is so named because they assume oversight of regulating both food and prescription medications.

Part IV – Communication and Patient Education

1. A
When communicating with another person, **gestures** emphasize an important point, **posture** can indicate either great interest or boredom, and **touch** can express encouragement or empathy.

2. D
A person who is **crossing their arms across their chest** may indicate the desire to place an unconscious barrier between themselves and others.

3. D
None of these statements are false.
Consistent eye contact can indicate a positive reaction to a speaker.
Consistent eye contact can indicate a lack of trust in the speaker.
The use of eye contact may be dependent on the culture of the listener.

4. C
The idea of mirroring body language to put people at ease is commonly used in interviews. Mirroring the body language of someone else indicates that they are understood.

5. C
The study of body language is called kinetic interpretation is false.

6. D
Nonverbal communication can signal a lack of interest or an unfriendly attitude, and can make therapeutic communication difficult to achieve.

7. B
If a patient asks a question and you do not know the answer, the best answer is always the most helpful. I.e. that you will assist them in finding the answer.

8. A
Facilitation is an important communication technique in which phrases such as "go on," please continue," and "tell me more" are used to encourage the patient.

9. B
Reflection involves repeating something the patient just said to gain more specific information and to show that you are paying attention.

10. A
The two goals of the technique of summarization are **to ensure that the information that you've collected is accurate and complete and to signal the end of the interview.**

11. B
Paraphrasing is restating something that a patient has said, usually in fewer words and with emphasis on the main points of their statement.

12. A
When **paraphrasing** is used in active listening, it demonstrates that you understand the patient's experience and allows them to evaluate their feeling by hearing them expressed by someone else.

13. A
The steps to attentive listening include, **maintaining eye contact and facing the person squarely.**

14. B
Facial expression, posture and tone of voice are elements of **nonverbal communication.**

15. D
Nonverbal communications can emphasize or contradict verbal messages is the only statement that is true.

16. C
Open-ended questions are used to obtain the most complete information available.

17. A
The statement, **an interviewer should never ask close-ended questions** is false. Closed-ended questions are appropriate in situations where a short answer, without elaboration is required.

18. C
Nodding provides encourages the patient to continue talking without indicating agreement or disagreement.

19. A
Using phrases that address a person's feelings, such as "You must be worried about your headaches," demonstrates **empathy.**

20. D.
Role-playing can be an effective way to communicate with children.

Part V – Insurance, Records and Bookkeeping

1. A
A health maintenance organization (HMO) is an organization that provides managed care for health insurance contracts as a liaison with health care providers (hospitals, doctors, etc.). The Health Maintenance Organization Act of 1973 required employers with 25 or more employees to offer federally certified HMO options if the employer offers traditional healthcare options. Unlike traditional indemnity insurance, an HMO covers only care rendered by those doctors and other professionals who have agreed to treat patients in accordance with the HMO's guidelines and restrictions in exchange for a steady stream of customers.[27]

2. A
In health insurance in the United States, a preferred

provider organization (or "PPO," sometimes called a participating provider organization or preferred provider option) is a managed care organization of medical doctors, hospitals, and other health care providers who have covenanted with an insurer or a third-party administrator to provide health care at reduced rates to the insurer's or administrator's clients.

A preferred provider organization is a subscription-based medical care arrangement. A membership allows a substantial discount below the regularly charged rates of the designated professionals partnered with the organization. Preferred provider organizations themselves earn money by charging an access fee to the insurance company for the use of their network (unlike the usual insurance with premiums and corresponding payments paid either in full or partially by the insurance provider to the medical doctor). They negotiate with providers to set fee schedules, and handle disputes between insurers and providers.[28]

3. B
TRICARE, formerly known as the Civilian Health and Medical Program of the Uniformed Services (CHAMPUS), is a health care program of the United States Department of Defense Military Health System. TRICARE provides civilian health benefits for military personnel, military retirees, and their dependents, including some members of the Reserve Component.[29]

4. D
Medicare is a social insurance program administered by the United States government, providing health insurance coverage to people who are aged 65 and over; to those who are under 65 and are permanently physically disabled or who have a congenital physical disability; or to those who meet other special criteria.[30]

5. B
Relative value units (RVUs) are a measure of value used in the Medicare reimbursement formula for physician services. RVUs are a part of the resource-based relative value scale (RBRVS).[31]

6. B
An insured person's child is a dependent.

7. C
Point of service is where the service is delivered. There is also a Point Of Service insurance plan where members of a POS plan do not make a choice about which system to use until the point at which they require the service.

8. B
Precertification, also knows as preauthorization. Most insurance companies require precertification 24 hours before a patient is admitted or undergoes certain procedures.

9. B
Major Medical, previously known as catastrophic coverage, is a type of insurance that covers large medical charges for catastrophic and/or long illness or conditions.

10. A
Part A covers inpatient hospital stays (at least overnight), including semiprivate room, food, and tests.

Part A covers brief stays for convalescence in a skilled nursing facility if certain criteria are met:

1. A preceding hospital stay must be at least three days, three midnights, not counting the discharge date.
2. The nursing home stay must be for something diagnosed during the hospital stay or for the main cause of hospital stay.
3. If the patient is not receiving rehabilitation but has some other ailment that requires skilled nursing supervision then the nursing home stay would be covered.

The nursing home must render skilled care. Medicare part A does not pay for custodial, non-skilled, or long-term care activities, including activities of daily living (ADL) such as personal hygiene, cooking, cleaning, etc.[30]

11. B
Part B is Medical Insurance for some services and products not covered by Part A, generally on an outpatient basis. Part

B is optional and the beneficiary may defer if they or their spouse is still working. There is a lifetime penalty (10% per year) imposed for not enrolling in Part B unless actively working. Part B coverage begins once a patient meets his or her deductible, then typically Medicare covers 80% of approved services, while patient pays the remaining 20%. Part B coverage includes physician and nursing services, x-rays, laboratory and diagnostic tests, influenza and pneumonia vaccinations, blood transfusions, renal dialysis, outpatient hospital procedures, limited ambulance transportation, immunosuppressive drugs for organ transplant recipients, chemotherapy, hormonal treatments such as Lupron, and other outpatient medical treatments administered in a doctor's office. Part B covers medication if a physician administers the medication during an office visit.

Part B also helps with durable medical equipment (DME), including canes, walkers, wheelchairs, and mobility scooters for those with mobility impairments. Prosthetic devices such as artificial limbs and breast prosthesis following mastectomy, as well as one pair of eyeglasses following cataract surgery, and oxygen for home use are also covered.[30]

12. A
TRICARE, formerly known as the Civilian Health and Medical Program of the Uniformed Services (CHAMPUS), is a health care program of the United States Department of Defence Military Health System. TRICARE provides civilian health benefits for military personnel, military retirees, and their dependents, including some members of the Reserve Component.[29]

13. B
Workers Compensation does not cover spouses. Workers' Compensation is a form of insurance providing wage replacement and medical benefits to employees injured in the course of employment in exchange for mandatory relinquishment of the employee's right to sue his or her employer for the tort of negligence. The compensation bargain is the trade-off between assured, limited coverage and lack of recourse outside the worker compensation system[32]

14. B
Resource-based relative value scale (RBRVS) is a schema used to determine how much money medical providers should be paid. Medicare partially uses the RBRVS as well as nearly all Health maintenance organizations (HMOs).

RBRVS assigns procedures performed by a physician or other medical provider a relative value that is adjusted by geographic region (so a procedure performed in Manhattan is worth more than a procedure performed in El Paso). This value is then multiplied by a fixed conversion factor, which changes annually, to determine the amount of payment.

RBRVS determines prices based on three separate factors: physician work (52%), practice expense (44%), and malpractice expense (4%).[33]

15. A
The Day Sheet is a daily record of services performed, charges and payments received.

16. C
The Day Sheet is an accounts receivable document.

17. B
The petty cash account is for small purchases.

Petty cash is a small amount of discretionary funds in the form of cash used for expenditures where it is not sensible to make any disbursement by cheque, because of the inconvenience and costs of writing, signing and then cashing the cheque. Petty cash is usually stored in a Petty Cash box and kept secure with a key.
The most common way of accounting for petty cash expenditures is to use the imprest system. The initial fund would be created by issuing a cheque for the desired amount. An amount of $100 would typically be sufficient for most small business needs as the expenses to be covered are for small amounts. The bookkeeping entry for this initial fund would be to debit Petty Cash and credit bank account.[34]

18. B
Accounts Payable is a file or account sub-ledger that records amounts that a person or company owes to suppliers, but has not paid yet (a form of debt), sometimes referred as trade payables. When the office receives an invoice, it is added to the file, and removed when it is paid. Thus, the A/P is a form of credit that suppliers offer to their customers by allowing them to pay for a product or service after it has already been received.[35]

19. C
A bill of lading (BL - sometimes called BOL or B/L) is a document issued by a carrier to a shipper, acknowledging that specified goods have been received on board as cargo for conveyance to a named place for delivery to the consignee. The term derives from the verb "to lade" which means to load a cargo onto a ship or other form of transportation.[36]

20. A
Accounts Receivable is money owed to a business by its clients (customers or patients) and shown on its Balance Sheet as an asset.

21. A
Superbill is itemized form utilized by healthcare providers for reflecting rendered services. Superbill is the main data source for creation of healthcare claim, which the office submits to payers (insurances, funds, programs) for reimbursement. Although the superbill form is not unified, and it is created/modified depending on healthcare provider specialty, type of rendered services, additional requirements, as well as ease of handling, there is a set of obligatory attributes, relevant to all superbill types.[37]

22. A
Debit and credit are the two aspects of every financial transaction. Their use and implication is the fundamental concept in the double-entry bookkeeping system, in which every debit transaction must have a corresponding credit transaction(s) and vice versa.

Debits and credits are a system of notation used in bookkeeping to determine how to record any financial transaction. In financial accounting or bookkeeping, "Dr" (Debit) means left side of a ledger account and "Cr" (Credit) is the right side of a ledger account.

23. D
Net income is the residual income of a firm after adding total revenue and gains and subtracting all expenses and losses for the reporting period.

24. B
A Bank reconciliation is a process that explains the difference between the bank balance shown in an organization's bank statement, as supplied by the bank, and the corresponding amount shown in the organization's own accounting records at a particular time.
Such differences may occur, for example, because

- a cheque issued by the organization has not been presented to the bank,
- a banking transaction, such as a credit received, or a charge made by the bank, has not yet been recorded in the organization's books
- either the bank or the organization itself has made an error

Part VI Fundamental Writing Skills

1. C
Comma separate phrases.

2. B
To travel around the globe, you have to drive 25,000 miles.

3. A
The dog loved chasing bones, but never ate them; it was running that he enjoyed.

4. B
The semicolon links independent clauses with a conjuction (therefore).

5. D
The third conditional is used for talking about an unreal situation (that did not happen) in the past. For example, "If I had studied harder, [if clause] I would have passed the exam [main clause]. Which is the same as, "I failed the exam, because I didn't study hard enough."

6. A
The third conditional is used for talking about an unreal situation (that did not happen) in the past. For example, "If I had studied harder, [if clause] I would have passed the exam [main clause]. Which is the same as, "I failed the exam, because I didn't study hard enough."

7. A
Disagreeing with a negative statement uses "neither."

8. C
Doesn't, does not, or does is used with the third person singular--words like he, she, and it. Don't, do not, or do is used for other subjects.

9. A
Bring vs. Take. Usage depends on your location. Something coming your way is brought to you. Something going away is taken from you.

10. C
Bring vs. Take. Usage depends on your location. Something coming your way is brought to you. Something going away is taken from you.

11. C
Fewer vs. Less. Fewer is used with countables and less is used with uncountables.

12. B
Fewer vs. Less. Fewer is used with countables and less is used with uncountables.

13. A
However Usage. "However" usually has a comma before and after.

14. D
However Usage. "However" usually has a comma before and after.

15. A
The third conditional is used for talking about an unreal situation (that did not happen) in the past. For example, "If I had studied harder, [if clause] I would have passed the exam [main clause]. Which is the same as, "I failed the exam, because I didn't study hard enough."

16. D
The third conditional is used for talking about an unreal situation (that did not happen) in the past. For example, "If I had studied harder, [if clause] I would have passed the exam [main clause]. Which is the same as, "I failed the exam, because I didn't study hard enough."

17. D
A vs. An. The article 'a' come before a consonant and 'an' comes before a vowel.

18. A
Accept vs. Except. To accept is to receive or to say yes. Except is a preposition that means excluding.

19. A
Advise vs. Advice. To advise is to give advice. Advice is an opinion that someone offers.

20. C
Adapt vs. Adopt.
Adapt means "to change." Usually we adapt to someone or something. Adopt means "to take as one's own."

21. D
Among vs. Between. Among is for more than 2 items, and between is only for 2 items.

When he's among friends (many or more than 2) Robert seems confident, but, between you and me (two) he is really very shy.

22. D
At vs. About. At refers to a specific time and about refers to a more general time. A common usage is 'at about 10,' but it isn't proper grammar.

23. B
Beside vs. Besides. Beside means next to, and besides means in addition to.

24. A
Can vs. May. Can refers to ability and may refers to permission.

Although John can swim (is able to. very well, he may not (permission. be allowed to swim in the pool.

25. B
Continual vs. Continuous. Continuous means a time with no interruption and continual means a time with interuption.

Her continual absences (with interuption – not always absent. caused a continuous disruption (the disruption was onging without interuption. at the office.

26. A
Emigrate vs. Immigrate. To emigrate means to leave one's country and to immigrate means to come to a country.

27. C
Further vs. Farther. Farther is used for physical distance, and further is used for figurative distance.

28. B
Former vs. Latter. Former refers to the first of two things, latter to the second.

29. A
Sit vs. Set. Set requires an object – something to set down. Sit is something that you do, like sit on the chair.

30. C
The names of God, specific deities, religious figures, and holy books are capitalized.

31. B
Capitalize a title when used with a name or other noun.

32. B
Titles preceding names are capitalized, but not titles that follow names.

33. C
Holidays are capitalized, the names of seasons are not.

Practice Test 2

The questions below are not the same as you will find on the CMA® - that would be too easy! And nobody knows what the questions will be and they change all the time. Below are general questions that cover the same subject areas as the CMA®. So, while the format and exact wording of the questions may differ slightly, and change from year to year, if you can answer the questions below, you will have no problem with the CMA®.

For the best results, take these Practice Test Questions as if it were the real exam. Set aside time when you will not be disturbed, and a location that is quiet and free of distractions. Read the instructions carefully, read each question carefully, and answer to the best of your ability.

Use the bubble answer sheets provided. When you have completed the Practice Questions, check your answer against the Answer Key and read the explanation provided.

Do not attempt more than one set of practice test questions in one day. After completing the first practice test, wait two or three days before attempting the second set of questions.

Part I – Medical Terminology

1. Ⓐ Ⓑ Ⓒ Ⓓ
2. Ⓐ Ⓑ Ⓒ Ⓓ
3. Ⓐ Ⓑ Ⓒ Ⓓ
4. Ⓐ Ⓑ Ⓒ Ⓓ
5. Ⓐ Ⓑ Ⓒ Ⓓ
6. Ⓐ Ⓑ Ⓒ Ⓓ
7. Ⓐ Ⓑ Ⓒ Ⓓ
8. Ⓐ Ⓑ Ⓒ Ⓓ
9. Ⓐ Ⓑ Ⓒ Ⓓ
10. Ⓐ Ⓑ Ⓒ Ⓓ
11. Ⓐ Ⓑ Ⓒ Ⓓ
12. Ⓐ Ⓑ Ⓒ Ⓓ
13. Ⓐ Ⓑ Ⓒ Ⓓ
14. Ⓐ Ⓑ Ⓒ Ⓓ
15. Ⓐ Ⓑ Ⓒ Ⓓ
16. Ⓐ Ⓑ Ⓒ Ⓓ
17. Ⓐ Ⓑ Ⓒ Ⓓ
18. Ⓐ Ⓑ Ⓒ Ⓓ
19. Ⓐ Ⓑ Ⓒ Ⓓ
20. Ⓐ Ⓑ Ⓒ Ⓓ
21. Ⓐ Ⓑ Ⓒ Ⓓ
22. Ⓐ Ⓑ Ⓒ Ⓓ
23. Ⓐ Ⓑ Ⓒ Ⓓ
24. Ⓐ Ⓑ Ⓒ Ⓓ
25. Ⓐ Ⓑ Ⓒ Ⓓ
26. Ⓐ Ⓑ Ⓒ Ⓓ
27. Ⓐ Ⓑ Ⓒ Ⓓ
28. Ⓐ Ⓑ Ⓒ Ⓓ
29. Ⓐ Ⓑ Ⓒ Ⓓ
30. Ⓐ Ⓑ Ⓒ Ⓓ
31. Ⓐ Ⓑ Ⓒ Ⓓ
32. Ⓐ Ⓑ Ⓒ Ⓓ
33. Ⓐ Ⓑ Ⓒ Ⓓ
34. Ⓐ Ⓑ Ⓒ Ⓓ
35. Ⓐ Ⓑ Ⓒ Ⓓ
36. Ⓐ Ⓑ Ⓒ Ⓓ
37. Ⓐ Ⓑ Ⓒ Ⓓ
38. Ⓐ Ⓑ Ⓒ Ⓓ
39. Ⓐ Ⓑ Ⓒ Ⓓ
40. Ⓐ Ⓑ Ⓒ Ⓓ
41. Ⓐ Ⓑ Ⓒ Ⓓ
42. Ⓐ Ⓑ Ⓒ Ⓓ
43. Ⓐ Ⓑ Ⓒ Ⓓ
44. Ⓐ Ⓑ Ⓒ Ⓓ
45. Ⓐ Ⓑ Ⓒ Ⓓ
46. Ⓐ Ⓑ Ⓒ Ⓓ
47. Ⓐ Ⓑ Ⓒ Ⓓ
48. Ⓐ Ⓑ Ⓒ Ⓓ
49. Ⓐ Ⓑ Ⓒ Ⓓ
50. Ⓐ Ⓑ Ⓒ Ⓓ
51. Ⓐ Ⓑ Ⓒ Ⓓ
52. Ⓐ Ⓑ Ⓒ Ⓓ
53. Ⓐ Ⓑ Ⓒ Ⓓ
54. Ⓐ Ⓑ Ⓒ Ⓓ
55. Ⓐ Ⓑ Ⓒ Ⓓ
56. Ⓐ Ⓑ Ⓒ Ⓓ
57. Ⓐ Ⓑ Ⓒ Ⓓ
58. Ⓐ Ⓑ Ⓒ Ⓓ
59. Ⓐ Ⓑ Ⓒ Ⓓ
60. Ⓐ Ⓑ Ⓒ Ⓓ

Part II – Anatomy and Physiology

1. A B C D
2. A B C D
3. A B C D
4. A B C D
5. A B C D
6. A B C D
7. A B C D
8. A B C D
9. A B C D
10. A B C D
11. A B C D
12. A B C D
13. A B C D
14. A B C D
15. A B C D
16. A B C D
17. A B C D
18. A B C D
19. A B C D
20. A B C D
21. A B C D
22. A B C D
23. A B C D
24. A B C D
25. A B C D
26. A B C D
27. A B C D
28. A B C D
29. A B C D
30. A B C D
31. A B C D
32. A B C D
33. A B C D
34. A B C D
35. A B C D
36. A B C D
37. A B C D
38. A B C D
39. A B C D
40. A B C D
41. A B C D
42. A B C D
43. A B C D
44. A B C D
45. A B C D
46. A B C D
47. A B C D
48. A B C D
49. A B C D
50. A B C D

Part III – Medical Law, Ethics and Legislation

1. Ⓐ Ⓑ Ⓒ Ⓓ
2. Ⓐ Ⓑ Ⓒ Ⓓ
3. Ⓐ Ⓑ Ⓒ Ⓓ
4. Ⓐ Ⓑ Ⓒ Ⓓ
5. Ⓐ Ⓑ Ⓒ Ⓓ
6. Ⓐ Ⓑ Ⓒ Ⓓ
7. Ⓐ Ⓑ Ⓒ Ⓓ
8. Ⓐ Ⓑ Ⓒ Ⓓ
9. Ⓐ Ⓑ Ⓒ Ⓓ
10. Ⓐ Ⓑ Ⓒ Ⓓ
11. Ⓐ Ⓑ Ⓒ Ⓓ
12. Ⓐ Ⓑ Ⓒ Ⓓ
13. Ⓐ Ⓑ Ⓒ Ⓓ
14. Ⓐ Ⓑ Ⓒ Ⓓ
15. Ⓐ Ⓑ Ⓒ Ⓓ
16. Ⓐ Ⓑ Ⓒ Ⓓ
17. Ⓐ Ⓑ Ⓒ Ⓓ
18. Ⓐ Ⓑ Ⓒ Ⓓ
19. Ⓐ Ⓑ Ⓒ Ⓓ
20. Ⓐ Ⓑ Ⓒ Ⓓ
21. Ⓐ Ⓑ Ⓒ Ⓓ
22. Ⓐ Ⓑ Ⓒ Ⓓ
23. Ⓐ Ⓑ Ⓒ Ⓓ
24. Ⓐ Ⓑ Ⓒ Ⓓ
25. Ⓐ Ⓑ Ⓒ Ⓓ
26. Ⓐ Ⓑ Ⓒ Ⓓ
27. Ⓐ Ⓑ Ⓒ Ⓓ
28. Ⓐ Ⓑ Ⓒ Ⓓ
29. Ⓐ Ⓑ Ⓒ Ⓓ
30. Ⓐ Ⓑ Ⓒ Ⓓ

Part IV – Communication and Patient Education

1. (A) (B) (C) (D)   11. (A) (B) (C) (D)
2. (A) (B) (C) (D)   12. (A) (B) (C) (D)
3. (A) (B) (C) (D)   13. (A) (B) (C) (D)
4. (A) (B) (C) (D)   14. (A) (B) (C) (D)
5. (A) (B) (C) (D)   15. (A) (B) (C) (D)
6. (A) (B) (C) (D)   16. (A) (B) (C) (D)
7. (A) (B) (C) (D)   17. (A) (B) (C) (D)
8. (A) (B) (C) (D)   18. (A) (B) (C) (D)
9. (A) (B) (C) (D)   19. (A) (B) (C) (D)
10. (A) (B) (C) (D)   20. (A) (B) (C) (D)

Part V – Insurance, Records and Bookkeeping

1. Ⓐ Ⓑ Ⓒ Ⓓ   11. Ⓐ Ⓑ Ⓒ Ⓓ   21. Ⓐ Ⓑ Ⓒ Ⓓ
2. Ⓐ Ⓑ Ⓒ Ⓓ   12. Ⓐ Ⓑ Ⓒ Ⓓ   22. Ⓐ Ⓑ Ⓒ Ⓓ
3. Ⓐ Ⓑ Ⓒ Ⓓ   13. Ⓐ Ⓑ Ⓒ Ⓓ   23. Ⓐ Ⓑ Ⓒ Ⓓ
4. Ⓐ Ⓑ Ⓒ Ⓓ   14. Ⓐ Ⓑ Ⓒ Ⓓ   24. Ⓐ Ⓑ Ⓒ Ⓓ
5. Ⓐ Ⓑ Ⓒ Ⓓ   15. Ⓐ Ⓑ Ⓒ Ⓓ
6. Ⓐ Ⓑ Ⓒ Ⓓ   16. Ⓐ Ⓑ Ⓒ Ⓓ
7. Ⓐ Ⓑ Ⓒ Ⓓ   17. Ⓐ Ⓑ Ⓒ Ⓓ
8. Ⓐ Ⓑ Ⓒ Ⓓ   18. Ⓐ Ⓑ Ⓒ Ⓓ
9. Ⓐ Ⓑ Ⓒ Ⓓ   19. Ⓐ Ⓑ Ⓒ Ⓓ
10. Ⓐ Ⓑ Ⓒ Ⓓ   20. Ⓐ Ⓑ Ⓒ Ⓓ

Part VI – Fundamental Writing Skills

1. Ⓐ Ⓑ Ⓒ Ⓓ
2. Ⓐ Ⓑ Ⓒ Ⓓ
3. Ⓐ Ⓑ Ⓒ Ⓓ
4. Ⓐ Ⓑ Ⓒ Ⓓ
5. Ⓐ Ⓑ Ⓒ Ⓓ
6. Ⓐ Ⓑ Ⓒ Ⓓ
7. Ⓐ Ⓑ Ⓒ Ⓓ
8. Ⓐ Ⓑ Ⓒ Ⓓ
9. Ⓐ Ⓑ Ⓒ Ⓓ
10. Ⓐ Ⓑ Ⓒ Ⓓ
11. Ⓐ Ⓑ Ⓒ Ⓓ
12. Ⓐ Ⓑ Ⓒ Ⓓ
13. Ⓐ Ⓑ Ⓒ Ⓓ
14. Ⓐ Ⓑ Ⓒ Ⓓ
15. Ⓐ Ⓑ Ⓒ Ⓓ
16. Ⓐ Ⓑ Ⓒ Ⓓ
17. Ⓐ Ⓑ Ⓒ Ⓓ
18. Ⓐ Ⓑ Ⓒ Ⓓ
19. Ⓐ Ⓑ Ⓒ Ⓓ
20. Ⓐ Ⓑ Ⓒ Ⓓ
21. Ⓐ Ⓑ Ⓒ Ⓓ
22. Ⓐ Ⓑ Ⓒ Ⓓ
23. Ⓐ Ⓑ Ⓒ Ⓓ
24. Ⓐ Ⓑ Ⓒ Ⓓ
25. Ⓐ Ⓑ Ⓒ Ⓓ
26. Ⓐ Ⓑ Ⓒ Ⓓ
27. Ⓐ Ⓑ Ⓒ Ⓓ
28. Ⓐ Ⓑ Ⓒ Ⓓ
29. Ⓐ Ⓑ Ⓒ Ⓓ
30. Ⓐ Ⓑ Ⓒ Ⓓ
31. Ⓐ Ⓑ Ⓒ Ⓓ
32. Ⓐ Ⓑ Ⓒ Ⓓ
33. Ⓐ Ⓑ Ⓒ Ⓓ
34. Ⓐ Ⓑ Ⓒ Ⓓ
35. Ⓐ Ⓑ Ⓒ Ⓓ

Section I – Medical Terminology

1. Bodily organs can sometimes adhere to the _____, a two-layered membrane lining the abdominal cavity and covering abdominal organs; when this occurs, the problem is corrected through surgical release of _____ adhesions.

    a. Bodily organs can sometimes adhere to the peritoneum, a two-layered membrane lining the abdominal cavity and covering abdominal organs; when this occurs, it the problem is corrected through surgical release of peritoneal adhesions.

    b. Bodily organs can sometimes adhere to the adipose tissue, a two-layered membrane lining the abdominal cavity and covering abdominal organs; when this occurs, the problem is corrected through surgical release of adipose adhesions.

    c. Bodily organs can sometimes adhere to the perumbilicus, a two-layered membrane lining the abdominal cavity and covering abdominal organs; when this occurs, the problem is   corrected through surgical release of perumbilicus adhesions.

    d. Bodily organs can sometimes adhere to the perilingual, a two-layered membrane lining the abdominal cavity and covering abdominal organs; when this occurs, the problem is   corrected through surgical release of perilingual adhesions.

2. A/an _____ allows a physician to obtain a small, representative sample of tissue for microscopic examination; this is usually done to establish a diagnosis.

    a. Laparoscopy

    b. Endarterectomy

    c. Biopsy

    d. CRT

3. Which surgery is indicated when part of the intestine protrudes into the groin?

    a. Inguinal hernia repair

    b. Colectomy

    c. Adhesion repair

    d. Prostatectomy

4. _____ are distended veins in the lower rectum or anus; a/an _____ is performed to relieve this condition.

    a. Mastoids are distended veins in the lower rectum or anus; a mastectomy is performed to relieve this condition.

    b. Flavonoids are distended veins in the lower rectum or anus; a flavonoidectomy is performed to relieve this condition.

    c. Hemorrhoids are distended veins in the lower rectum or anus; a hemorrhoidectomy is performed to relieve this condition.

    d. Tumoroids are distended veins in the lower rectum or anus; a tumorectomy is performed to relieve this condition.

5. During _____, a tight band of transverse fibrous tissue is cut, releasing pressure on the median nerves and relieving symptoms.

    a. Adhesion repair surgery

    b. Open carpal tunnel surgery

    c. Carotid surgery

    d. Ligament surgery

6. A surgical procedure that unblocks the arteries located in the neck which supply blood to the brain is a/an _____.

   a. Carotid endarterectomy

   b. Arterial cleanse

   c. Peripheral endarterectomy

   d. Colectomy

7. _____ involves removal of the opaque contents of a lens of the eye via ultrasound waves, although, in some cases, the entire lens is removed and replaced with an artificial lens.

   a. Vitrectomy surgery

   b. Retinopathy surgery

   c. Laser surgery

   d. Cataract surgery

8. Which, if any, of the following statements concerning hysterectomies are false?

   a. A hysterectomy is the surgical removal of the uterus.

   b. A hysterectomy can be performed through either an abdominal incision or vaginally.

   c. Following a radical hysterectomy, a small number of patients are placed on a hormone replacement regimen.

   d. A radical hysterectomy includes the removal of the uterus, tubes, ovaries, adjacent lymph nodes and a portion of the vagina.

9. Which, if any, of the following statements about fluoroscopy are false?

   a. Fluoroscopy utilizes a continuous or pulsed bean of low-dose radiation.

   b. Fluoroscopy is a type of x-ray that can be used to evaluate the flow of blood through the arteries.

   c. Fluoroscopy produces a series of still images of the body part being examined.

   d. Images can be videotaped or sent to a monitor for viewing.

10. A/an _____ is a test employed to identify blockages in the circulatory system, diagnose stroke and determine the size and location of brain tumors and aneurysms.

   a. Angiogram

   b. Arterial fluid analysis

   c. Ultrasound imaging

   d. None of the above.

11. During a _____, a small sample of tissue is removed, usually under local anesthetic, examined microscopically for the purpose of diagnosis.

   a. Amniocentesis

   b. Biopsy

   c. Cerebrospinal analysis

   d. Culture

12. What areas of dysfunction are diagnosed through the use of electromyography?

a. Nerve and muscle dysfunction and spinal cord disease

b. Balance disorders and hearing loss

c. Arrhythmia and tachycardia

d. None of the above

13. Which, if any, of the following statements about cerebrospinal fluid analysis (CSF) are false?

a. CSF are tests that measure proteins, glucose and other chemicals contained in the fluid that protects the brain and spinal cord.

b. A lumbar puncture is performed to obtain a fluid sample, a painless procedure completed without the use of anesthetic.

c. CSF analysis can be used to diagnose infections (such as meningitis) and brain or spinal cord damage, as well as to measure intracranial pressure.

d. Some cases of multiple sclerosis can be detected through CSF.

14. _____, also known as a _____, is used to detect bone and vascular anomalies, certain types of brain tumors, and blood clots in patients who have experienced a stroke or brain damage due to an injury.

a. Electroencephalography, EEG

b. Electromyography, EMG

c. Positron emission tomography, PET

d. Computed tomography, CT scan

15. Using the magnetic properties of the blood, a _____ produces real-time images of blood flow to certain areas of the brain and assesses damage due to head injury or disorders such as Alzheimer's disease.

    a. Positron emission tomography

    b. Ultrasound imaging

    c. Electroencephalography

    d. Functional MRI (fMRI)

16. Which, if any, of the following statements about positron emission tomography (PET) scans are false?

    a. Prior to the test, a low-level radioactive isotope is injected into the patient's bloodstream.

    b. PET scans are used to detect tumors and measure cellular metabolism.

    c. PET scans are frequently used instead of CT or MRI scans, which are significantly less accurate.

    d. Alterations in the brain as a result of damage or drug use can be determined through the use of a PET scan.

17. The goal of _____, also called physiatry, is to enhance and restore functional ability to those with disabilities or physical impairments.

    a. Rheumatology

    b. Physical medicine and rehabilitation

    c. Orthopedic medicine

    d. Immunology

18. _____ is a branch of medicine concerned with diseases of the rectum, anus, colon and pelvic floor.

    a. Urology

    b. Nephrology

    c. Immunology

    d. Proctology

19. Which, of any, of the following statement concerning pulmonology are true?

    a. Pulmonology is also referred to as pneumology.

    b. The focus of this specialty is the diagnosis of lung diseases, as well as the prevention of secondary diseases such as tuberculosis.

    c. Pulmonology is closely associated with critical care medicine in that it deals with patients who require mechanical ventilation.

    d. All of the above.

20. Which branch of medicine centers around the treatment of conditions affecting joints, muscles, and bones, as well as some autoimmune diseases and vasculitis?

    a. Immunology

    b. Rheumatology

    c. Angiology

    d. Rehabilitative medicine

21. _____ medicine, known in Europe as angiology, is a medical specialty centered on the study of the _____ and _____ systems and diseases associated with those systems.

    a. Vascular medicine, known in Europe as angiology, is a medical specialty centered on the study of the circulatory and lymphatic systems and diseases associated with those systems.

    b. Thoracic medicine, known in Europe as angiology, is a medical specialty centered on the study of the circulatory and lymphatic systems and diseases associated with those systems.

    c. Vascular medicine, known in Europe as angiology, is a medical specialty centered on the study of the respiratory and circulatory systems and diseases associated with those systems.

    d. Physical medicine, known in Europe as angiology, is a medical specialty centered on the study of the circulatory and lymphatic systems and diseases associated with those systems.

22. Which, if any, of the following statements about thoracic surgery are false?

    a. Thoracic surgeons treat diseases that affect the organs within the chest.

    b. Treatment most frequently involves conditions of the lungs, chest wall and diaphragm.

    c. Many times, thoracic surgery is grouped with cardiac surgery and termed cardiothoracic surgery.

    d. All of these statements are true.

23. _____ is both a medical and surgical specialty focused on the urinary tracts of both men and women and the reproductive systems of males.

    a. Nephrology
    b. Urology
    c. Andrology
    d. Endocrinology

24. _____ surgery is surgery performed on the heart and/or major blood vessels to treat complications of ischemic heart disease, correct congenital heart disease, etc.

    a. Cardiothoracic
    b. Angiologic
    c. Cardiovascular
    d. Transplant

25. The Greek prefix gastro-, in a medical context, means

    a. the intestines.
    b. the bladder.
    c. the lungs.
    d. the stomach.

26. The Greek prefix gluco-, in a medical context, means

    a. sour.
    b. bitter.
    c. sweet.
    d. bland.

27. The prefix glyco-, means

   a. salt.
   b. sugar.
   c. perspiration.
   d. medicine.

28. The Latin prefix halluc-, in a medical context means

   a. hearing things that aren't there.
   b. experiencing pain long after the event.
   c. wandering mind.
   d. forgetting things.

29. The Greek prefix hemi-, in a medical context means

   a. one-third.
   b. one-half.
   c. one fourth.
   d. one tenth.

30. The Latin prefix huero- has come to mean pertaining to:

   a. the lower leg.
   b. the calf
   c. the wrist.
   d. the upper arm or shoulder.

31. The Greek prefix hydro-, in a medical context, means

   a. air
   b. dust.
   c. water.
   d. helium.

32. The Greek prefix hyper-, in a medical context, means

    a. something that is slow.

    b. something that is normal.

    c. something that is extreme or which is beyond normal.

    d. something that can fly.

33. The Greek prefix hypo-, in a medical context, means

    a. something that is slow.

    b. something that is normal.

    c. something that is below normal.

    d. something that is extreme.

34. The Latin prefix infra-, in a medical context, means

    a. above.

    b. below.

    c. in between.

    d. around.

35. The Latin prefix intra-, in a medical context, means

    a. within.

    b. outside of.

    c. above.

    d. below.

36. The Greek prefix kerato-, in a medical context, means

    a. nose membrane.

    b. cornea, eye or skin.

    c. hearing or within the ear.

    d. inside the brain.

37. The Greek suffix -ac, in a medical context, means

   a. away from.
   b. pertaining to.
   c. unlike.
   d. distant.

38. The Greek suffix -acusis, in a medical context, means

   a. of or for the sense of smell.
   b. of or for the sense of taste.
   c. of or for the sense of hearing.
   d. of or for the sense of sight.

39. The Greek suffix -ase, in a medical context, means

   a. unity.
   b. division.
   c. entropy.
   d. good health.

40. The Greek suffix -cele, in a medical context, means

   a. division.
   b. collecting.
   c. disease.
   d. pouching; hernia.

41. The Greek suffix, centesis, in a medical context, means

   a. an operation that does not require stitches.
   b. a surgical puncture for aspiration.
   c. a doctor who works on the eyes.
   d. one hundred.

42. The Latin suffix -cidal means

a. bringing new life.
b. putting to sleep.
c. making someone ill.
d. destroying or killing.

43. The Greek suffix -desis, in a medical context, means

a. binding.
b. loosening.
c. limber.
d. ten or more.

44. The suffix -dynia, in a medical context, means

a. pain.
b. pain relief.
c. terminal illness.
d. instantaneous healing.

45. The Greek suffix -ectomy, in a medical context, means

a. a disease of the appendix.
b. surgery to remove either a body part or a portion of a body part.
c. surgery on the tonsils.
d. chemicals used to put a person to sleep during an operation.

46. The Greek suffix -emia, in a medical context, means

a. a condition of the blood.
b. a condition of the heart.
c. a condition of the eyes.
d. a condition of the lungs.

47. The Greek suffix -ist, in a medical context, means

 a. a doctor with little experience.
 b. a vapor.
 c. one who specializes
 d. one who studies under someone else.

48. The suffix -itis, in a medical context, means

 a. a bacterial disease.
 b. a blood disorder.
 c. brittleness of the bones.
 d. an inflammation.

49. The Greek suffix -lepsy, in a medical context, means

 a. a fatal disease.
 b. a condition of the lungs.
 c. mental disability.
 d. an attack or seizure.

50. The Greek suffix -logy means

 a. study.
 b. time.
 c. a written diary.
 d. arthritis.

51. The Greek suffix -meter means

 a. something used to make an incision.
 b. something used to count or measure.
 c. something used on the grass.
 d. something used to diagnose tooth or mouth disease.

52. The Greek suffix -oid means

   a. mechanical in nature.

   b. being totally unlike something else.

   c. resembling something else.

   d. human emotions in a non-human organism.

53. The Greek suffix -oma or -omata, in a medical context, means

   a. a large bone.

   b. a fruit that resembles a vegetable.

   c. an invisible organism.

   d. a mass or tumor.

54. The Greek suffix -osis, in a medical context, means

   a. a decrease or cure.

   b. an increase or condition.

   c. hypnotic state.

   d. like paradise; perfect.

55. The Greek suffix -pathy, in a medical context, means

   a. a disease or disorder.

   b. a cure or healing.

   c. a road or course.

   d. pertaining to the bones.

56. The Greek suffix -plasty, in a medical context, means

   a. pasty or glue-like substance.

   b. occurring years ago.

   c. living tissue that resembles plastic.

   d. reconstruction or surgical repair.

57. The Greek suffix -rrhage means

a. declining.
b. bursting forth.
c. lowering.
d. deteriorating.

58. The Latin suffix, -tension, in a medical context, means

a. athletic ability.
b. communication ability.
c. pressure.
d. forgetful.

59. What does the medical abbreviation AED mean?

a. Automated External Defibrillator
b. Anatomical Exhibit Device
c. Alexander Entropy Discussion
d. Automated Exhibiting Defibrillator

60. What does the medical abbreviation a.c. mean?

a. After Completion.
b. Before Meals.
c. After Meals.
d. Before Bed.

Section II – Anatomy and Physiology

1. What is osteoporosis?

a. A brain disorder that moves to the leg bones.
b. A condition in which nerves become fragile.
c. An ailment in which muscles deteriorate.
d. An ailment in which bones become fragile because of loss of tissue

2. Marfan syndrome is an example of an ailment that, rather than affecting the bones themselves, afflicts _____.

a. the muscles.
b. the nerves.
c. the heart.
d. the connective tissue.

3. Which system would you describe as the blood distribution system?

a. Digestive system.
b. Musculoskeletal system.
c. Endocrine system.
d. Circulatory system

4. _____ are examples of nutrients passed along via the circulatory system.

a. Citric acids
b. Amino acids
c. Proteins
d. Nuclei

5. Other than blood, what else moves through the circulatory system?

   a. Traces of bone
   b. Sweat
   c. Lymph
   d. Mercury

6. What are the main components of the circulatory system?

   a. The heart, veins and blood vessels.
   b. The heart, brain, and ears.
   c. The nose, throat and ears.
   d. The lungs, stomach, and kidneys.

7. Which disease of the circulatory system is one of the most frequent causes of death in North America?

   a. The cold
   b. Pneumonia
   c. Arthritis
   d. Heart disease

8. One disease of the circulatory system, which is often mistakenly thought to be a heart attack, is _____.

   a. Cardiac arrest
   b. High blood pressure
   c. Angina
   d. Acid reflux

9. What is a more common name for the circulatory system disease known as hypertension?

    a. Anemia

    b. High blood pressure

    c. Angina

    d. Cardiac arrest

10. A condition in which the heart beats too fast, too slow, or with an irregular beat is called _____.

    a. Hypertension

    b. Angina

    c. Cardiac arrest

    d. Arrythmia

11. What is the respiratory system?

    a. The system that brings oxygen into the body and expels carbon dioxide from the body.

    b. The system that sends blood to and from the heart.

    c. The system that processes food that enters the body.

    d. The system that expels urine from the body.

12. Which of the following is an example of an important component of the respiratory system?

    a. The cornea

    b. The lungs

    c. The kidneys

    d. The stomach

13. The exchange of oxygen for carbon dioxide takes place in the alveolar area of _____.

    a. the throat.

    b. the ears.

    c. the appendix.

    d. the lungs.

14. The part of the body that initiates inhalation is _____.

    a. the lungs.

    b. the diaphragm.

    c. the larynx.

    d. the kidneys.

15. Exhalation is often accomplished by _____.

    a. abdominal muscles

    b. chest muscles.

    c. the oesophagus.

    d. the nasal passageway.

16. What is the primary thing oxygenated through the work of the respiratory system?

    a. The brain

    b. The limbs

    c. The heart

    d. The blood

17. An example of an important side-benefit of the respiratory system is

    a. the air allows whistling.

    b. the oxygen expelled can be recycled for other uses.

    c. the air expelled from the mouth allows for speaking.

    d. the air expelled from the body also expels disease and germs.

18. An example of a lung disease caused or made worse by smoking is _____.

    a. emphysema.

    b. strep throat.

    c. muscular dystrophy.

    d. leukemia.

19. The immune system is _____.

    a. the system that expels waste from the body.

    b. the system that expels carbon dioxide from the body.

    c. the system that protects the body from disease and infection.

    d. the system that circulates blood through the body.

20. How does the immune system fight off disease?

    a. By identifying and killing tumor cells and pathogens.

    b. By creating new blood cells that fight disease.

    c. By expelling infection through the blood stream.

    d. By giving you energy to resist disease infections.

21. An example of a pathogen that the immune system detects is _____.

    a. an atom.
    b. a molecule.
    c. a vitamin.
    d. a virus.

22. Detection of pathogens can be complicated because _____.

    a. they evolve so quickly.
    b. they die so quickly.
    c. they are invisible.
    d. they multiply so quickly.

23. One of the best-known disorders that attack the immune system is _____.

    a. rabies
    b. hiv (the virus that causes aids)
    c. lung cancer
    d. muscular dystrophy

24. The process by which the immune system adapts over time to be more efficient in recognizing pathogens is known as _____.

    a. Acquired immunity
    b. AIDS
    c. Pathogens
    d. Acquired deficiency

25. _____ is an example of an early response by the immune system to infection.

    a. inhalation
    b. inflammation
    c. respiration
    d. exhalation.

26. Which cells are important weapons in the fight against infection?

    a. Red blood cells
    b. White blood cells
    c. Barrier cells
    d. Virus cells

27. What is the primary purpose of the digestive system?

    a. To expel food and liquids from the body.
    b. To absorb oxygen from food.
    c. To help circulate blood throughout the body.
    d. To convert food into a form that can provide nourishment for the body.

28. An important element in the digestive process is the _____ that help break down the food.

    a. Digestive juices
    b. Proteins
    c. Amino acids
    d. Chromosomes

29. Where does digestion begin?

    a. In the throat.
    b. In the stomach.
    c. In the intestines.
    d. In the mouth.

30. Which of these is not an example of a function of the stomach in digestion?

    a. Storing food.
    b. Cleansing food of impurities.
    c. Mixing food with digestive juices.
    d. Transferring food into the intestines.

31. What type of food stays in the stomach longest?

    a. Fats
    b. Proteins
    c. Carbohydrates
    d. Vitamins

32. One common digestive affliction that most people suffer at one time or other is _____.

    a. stomach cancer
    b. ulceritis
    c. indigestion
    d. the flu

33. When a pouch in the large intestine becomes inflamed, this becomes an affliction known as _____.

  a. diverticulosis
  b. diverticulitis
  c. acid reflux
  d. colon cancer

34. The best way to avoid most digestive diseases is _____.

  a. eating a healthy diet.
  b. eating only proteins.
  c. never eating dessert.
  d. trying not to get angry.

35. The three functions of the urinary system are _____.

  a. taking in oxygen, distributing oxygen, and helping the heart to relax.
  b. cleansing the blood stream, sending blood throughout the body, and fighting disease.
  c. improving lung function, improving stomach function and improving the heart rate.
  d. producing, storing and eliminating urine.

36. What is mostly true of urine?

  a. It's mostly comprised of healthy vitamins and nutrients.
  b. It's mostly comprised of waste material after the body has taken the nutrients from food and absorbed the water it needs.
  c. It's mostly useless in the body.
  d. It's mostly carbohydrates.

37. _____ is the name of the waste removed from the body through urine.

    a. urea

    b. urinalysis

    c. feces

    d. fat

38. One example of the blood stream's part in the digestive system is _____.

    a. preventing infection.

    b. carrying urea to the kidneys.

    c. expelling the urea from the body.

    d. the blood stream has no part in the digestive system.

39. Besides the kidney, the other major organ that takes part in the body's urinary system is _____.

    a. the penis

    b. the liver

    c. the stomach

    d. the bladder

40. Which of these describes the bladder?

    a. A pea-sized, circular organ.

    b. A balloon shaped, muscular organ.

    c. A square-ish organ about the size of the small intestine.

    d. A triangular organ exactly the same size as the heart.

41. What is a serious and common urinary disorder?

a. liver failure
b. stomach ulcer
c. kidney failure
d. lung cancer

42. The involuntary passage of urine defines the urinary-system disorder known as _____.

a. incontinence
b. impotence
c. bladder cancer
d. stomach ulcer

43. The lymphatic system is defined as the system which _____.

a. carries a clear liquid ("lymph") toward the heart.
b. carries a clear liquid ("lymph") out through the bowels.
c. heals the lymph nodes.
d. cleanses the blood stream of bacteria.

44. Which of these is true of lymphoid tissue?

a. It exists only in the lymph nodes.
b. It exists in many organs, although it's predominantly in the lymph nodes.
c. Humans have evolved beyond having lymphoid tissue in their bodies.
d. Lymphoid tissue is always cancerous.

45. What organ plays a big role in the lymphatic system?

    a. The spine.
    b. The kidney.
    c. The spleen.
    d. The liver.

46. What is a benefit of the lymphatic system?

    a. It has no known benefit.
    b. It removes most cancerous material from the body.
    c. It removes urine and feces from the body.
    d. It absorbs and transports fats and fatty acids from the body's circulatory system.

47. Which of these defines "metastasis?"

    a. Process of carrying cancer cells between various parts of the body.
    b. Process of eliminating all cancer cells.
    c. Process of expelling bodily waste from the body.
    d. Process in which a benign tumor becomes cancerous.

48. What is a common affliction of the lymphatic system?

    a. disintegration of the lymph nodes.
    b. swelling of the lymph nodes.
    c. constipation
    d. ear and nose problems.

49. An example of a cause of lymph node swelling is _____.

    a. infectious mononucleosis ("mono")
    b. the flu
    c. arthritis
    d. appendicitis

50. Another, more serious, example of a cause of lymph node swelling is _____.

    a. Tuberculosis
    b. Muscular dystrophy
    c. Multiple sclerosis
    d. Cancer

Section III – Medical Law, Ethics and Legislation

1. As a/an _____, you are required by law to report the abuse or neglect of a child, despite the fact that such a report breaches confidentiality.

    a. Third party
    b. Concerned citizen
    c. Mandated reporter
    d. Impartial witness

2. Signs of physical child abuse include:

    a. Flinching at sudden movements
    b. Non-attachment to parent
    c. Poor hygiene
    d. Sudden changes in weight or appetite

3. Signs of emotional abuse include:

a. Non-attachment to parent
b. Seductive behavior
c. Poor hygiene
d. Clothing inappropriate for the season

4. Signs of sexual abuse include:

a. Problems sitting or walking
b. Running away from home
c. Pregnancy or STD under the age of 14
d. All of the above

5. _____ is a pattern of not caring for a child, either physically or emotionally, that threatens the child's well-being.

a. Sexual abuse
b. Emotional abuse
c. Physical abuse
d. Child neglect

6. Fetal abuse has become an important and highly publicized issue in recent years. Which, if any, of the following are indications of fetal abuse?

a. Poor fetal growth on abdomen measurements or ultrasound
b. History or signs of domestic abuse
c. History or signs of maternal alcohol or drug use
d. All of the above

7. Which of the following statements are used by the Uniform Determination of Death Act (UDDA) to define death?

    a. The individual has sustained irreversible cessation of circulatory and respiratory functions.

    b. The individual has sustained irreversible cessation of all functions of the entire brain, including the brain stem.

    c. The person has lost their capacity for reasoning, self-awareness, communication, agency, and consciousness of the external world.

    d. Both a. and b.

8. _____ is defined as performing an act that one should not do at all or the unjust performance of such an act.

    a. Malpractice

    b. Malfeasance

    c. Misdemeanor

    d. A Lapse in judgment

9. According to the Health Information Portability and Accountability Act (HIPAA), which, if any, of these persons/organizations are allowed limited or full access to a patient's medical records?

    a. Family, even if the patient is fully competent and in charge of their affairs

    b. Close personal friends or life partners

    c. Government agencies such as Medicare, Workers Compensation and Social Security Disability Insurance

    d. None of the above

10. Under which of the following conditions, if any, can the medical information of a person at risk for HIV be released without patient permission?

    a. In an emergency situation to medical personnel or a court order has been issued

    b. For the purpose of review board approved research

    c. If the spouse has requested the information

    d. Unless patient permission has been given, medical information cannot be released under any conditions.

11. _____ _____ refers to what society owes a person in proportion to their individual needs and responsibilities, the resources available and society's responsibilities to the common good.

    a. Ethical distribution

    b. Distributive justice

    c. Benevolent justice

    d. Egalitarian ethics

12. A system of health care in which patients agree to visit only certain doctors and hospitals, and in which the cost of treatment is monitored is called _____.

    a. Managed care

    b. Private care

    c. Medicaid and Medicare

    d. Socialized medicine

13. Which of these statements regarding the medical treatment of illegal immigrants are true?

    a. In the United States, healthcare is not rationed by citizenship.

    b. The Illegal Immigration Reform and Immigrant Responsibility Act states that illegal immigrants are forbidden from receiving healthcare through Medicaid and Medicare with the exception of pregnancy care.

    c. The use of citizenship to ration healthcare violates the principle of benevolence.

    d. None of these statements are true.

14. A _____ indicates that a patient does not want cardiopulmonary resuscitation or defibrillation at the end of life, while a _____ order indicates that the patient rejects the use of a breathing tube in cases of respiratory arrest. _____ can be _____ at any time.

    a. A living will indicates that a patient does not want cardiopulmonary resuscitation or defibrillation at the end of life, while a DNI order indicates that the patient rejects the use of a breathing tube in cases of respiratory arrest. Both can be revoked at any time.

    b. A Do Not Resuscitate (DNR) indicates that a patient does not want cardiopulmonary resuscitation or defibrillation at the end of life while a DNI order indicates that the patient rejects the use of a breathing tube in cases of respiratory arrest. Neither can be revoked at any time.

    c. A Do Not Resuscitate (DNR) indicates that a patient does not want cardiopulmonary resuscitation or defibrillation at the end of life, while a DNI order indicates that the patient rejects the use of a breathing tube in cases of respiratory arrest. Both can be revoked at any time.

    d. A DNI order indicates that a patient does not want cardiopulmonary resuscitation or defibrillation at the end of life while a Do Not Resuscitate (DNR) indicates that the patient rejects the use of a breathing tube in cases of respiratory arrest. Both can be revoked at any time.

15. _____ is a legal term meaning that the patient has the mental and legal ability to make decisions.

   a. Autonomy
   b. Fitness
   c. Competence
   d. Common sense

16. In the United States, _____ refers to legal actions that cannot result in a person being punished by imprisonment.

   a. Criminal law
   b. Civil law
   c. Cause of action
   d. Comparative negligence

17. _____ refers to an ability to interact effectively with people of different _____.

   a. Religious aptitude refers to an ability to interact effectively with people of different faiths.
   b. Cultural diversity refers to an ability to interact effectively with people of different cultures.
   c. Ethnic forbearance refers to an ability to interact effectively with people of different ethnicities.
   d. Cultural competence refers to an ability to interact effectively with people of different cultures.

18. _____ are the most common type of treatment error.

   a. Medication errors
   b. Surgical errors
   c. Improper uses of medical equipment
   d. Misinterpretations of lab results

19. Types of medication errors include:

a. Administration errors which occur when the provider gives the wrong medicine to the patient

b. Pharmacy fulfillment errors

c. Transcription errors which occur when the pharmacist misreads the prescription or it is written incorrectly

d. All of the above

20. Which, if any, of the following statements about ethics and legality are true?

a. The law demands that patients are treated compassionately, while ethics require competent medical practice according to current standards and frequently exceed legal standards.

b. Breaches of ethics are usually not legally enforceable.

c. Ethics set rigid conduct standards that must be met while laws set flexible guidelines for conduct.

d. None of the above are true.

21. According to the tenets of the Americans with Disabilities Act, a medical professional cannot:

a. Charge excessively high fees.

b. Refuse to respond in emergency situations.

c. Terminate patient care in the middle of treatment.

d. Refuse to treat a patient with an infectious disease.

22. _____ is a federal law intended to standardize healthcare information and its use in the United States.

a. The Americans with Disabilities Act

b. The AMT Code of Ethics

c. The Health Information Portability and Accountability Act

d. The Protected Health Information Act

23. Which, if any, of the following statements about the patient rights of adolescents is true?

a. All 50 states allow minors to be tested for STDs, including HIV, without parental permission.

b. Informed consent forms must be written at the minor's level.

c. Adolescents must always obtain parental permission before placing a child for adoption.

d. In most states, minors may apply to a judge for a confidential alteration, which allows them to obtain an abortion without parental consent or notification.

24. An emancipated minor:

a. Is a person who, although not having reached the statutory age of majority, is granted the legal status of an adult

b. Is an adolescent who given birth to a child.

c. Can be living with and supported by their parents.

d. Has received approval for the action from their guardians.

25. A _____ is a person who has a duty to act primarily for another's benefit, as a trustee; this phrase also pertains the good faith and confidence involved in such a relationship.

a. Fiduciary

b. Guardian

c. Advocate

d. Sponsor

26. Which United States agency oversees the FDA?

    a. The U.S. Attorney General's Office.

    b. The Department of Education.

    c. OSHA.

    d. The United States Department of Health and Human Services.

27. The FDA is responsible for promoting health through regulating and supervising food safety, dietary supplements, pharmaceutical drugs and what else?

    a. Clothing.

    b. Livestock feed.

    c. Tobacco.

    d. Illegal marijuana plants.

28. Which of the following is not regulated by the FDA?

    a. Vaccines.

    b. Laundry detergent.

    c. Electromagnetic radiation.

    d. Medical devices.

29. Which person leads the FDA?

    a. The Commissioner of Food & Drugs.

    b. The Attorney General.

    c. The EPA Chairman.

    d. The U.S. Vice President.

30. ADA, when referring to the 1990s law that covers Americans with disabilities, stands for:

    a. Agency for Disabled Americans.

    b. Americans with Disabilities Act.

    c. America Dares to Act.

    d. American Defence Agency.

Section IV – Communication Skills and Patient Education

1. Which of the following can act as a barrier to communication?

    a. Attention

    b. Level of education

    c. Families

    d. Age

2. _____ is the zone around each person reserved for _____ and can vary according to _____.

    a. Personal space is the zone around each person reserved for conversation and can vary according to culture.

    b. Intimate space is the zone around each person reserved for conversation and can vary according to culture.

    c. Personal space is the zone around each person reserved for conversation and can vary according to age.

    d. Inner space is the zone around each person reserved for conversation and can vary according to culture.

3. When dealing with elderly patients, always _____.

   a. use their first names to establish intimacy.

   b. direct your questions to their caregivers.

   c. speak loudly and distinctly.

   d. address them as miss, mrs., or mr., followed by their last name.

4. A complete medical history should include:

   a. Insurance information

   b. The chief complaint

   c. Marital history

   d. All of the above

5. When documenting a patient's chief complaint, be careful to _____.

   a. Use the appropriate medical terms.

   b. Base your notes on comments from the family.

   c. Use the patient's exact words.

   d. None of the above.

6. Physical barriers to communication include:

   a. Time

   b. Environment

   c. Illness

   d. All of the above

7. If a patient does not seem to understand a question:

    a. Repeat the question using simpler terms.

    b. Ask them if they understood the question.

    c. Skip the question and come back to it later.

    d. Base your note on their medical history.

8. The interviewer says, "I want to be sure that I understand what you've said. You've been having headaches for several weeks, but you thought they would just go away on their own." The interviewer is using the interview technique of _____.

    a. Summarizing

    b. Paraphrasing

    c. Edifying

    d. Perception checking

9. For patients who are depressed, cognitively impaired, or unable to deal with complex communication at that particular moment, using _____ that require short answers can help obtain information.

    a. Indirect questions

    b. Feedback

    c. Direct questions

    d. Paraphrasing

10. Which, if any, of the following statements about the issue of silence during an interview are false?

a. While beneficial to the interview process, silence can sometimes be perceived as a lack of interest.

b. Silence should always be avoided in the interview process.

c. Silence allows the patient to think about their answer to a question.

d. Silence can be broken by short comments that do not require a response.

11. "You've been feeling depressed, haven't you?" is an example of a/an _____.

a. Indirect question

b. Direct question

c. Leading question

d. Feedback

12. Leading questions are an ineffective means of obtaining information because:

a. The patient may feel forced to give the answer the interviewer is looking for.

b. The patient may not understand the question.

c. The response is likely to be either short or unclear.

d. Asking a leading question is illegal.

13. During the interview process, the most accurate information is provided by _____.

a. Medical records

b. Family members

c. Close friends

d. The patient

14. When interviewing a patient with a hearing loss, remember to _____.

 a. Speak slowly and look directly at the patient.

 b. Ensure that the room is brightly lit.

 c. Write down your questions and have them write their answers.

 d. Both a) and b).

15. _____ is the key means of communication between healthcare workers.

 a. Email

 b. The telephone

 c. Conversation

 d. The medical record

16. A/an _____ is used to obtain _____ information and learn about past and current health problems.

 a. An interview is used to obtain insurance information and learn about past and current health problems.

 b. A health history is used to obtain subjective information and learn about past and current health problems.

 c. A biography is used to obtain sufficient information and learn about past and current health problems.

 d. A diagnostic procedure is used to obtain subjective information and learn about past and current health problems.

17. What is the first area to be covered when obtaining a health history?

 a. Chief complaint

 b. Insurance coverage

 c. Biographic information

 d. Family history

18. Using neutral remarks such as, "I see" and "I hear what you're saying" indicate _____ to the patient.

   a. Empathy

   b. Recognition

   c. Understanding

   d. Avoidance

19. In addition to providing _____ patient information to other healthcare professionals, it is necessary that one be able to _____ what others have added to the medical record.

   a. In addition to providing objective patient information to other healthcare professionals, it is necessary that one be able to increase what others have added to the medical record.

   b. In addition to providing legible patient information to other healthcare professionals, it is necessary that one be able to read what others have added to the medical record.

   c. In addition to providing accurate patient information to other healthcare professionals, it is necessary that one be able to discuss what others have added to the medical record.

   d. In addition to providing accurate patient information to other healthcare professionals, it is necessary that one be able to interpret what others have added to the medical record.

20. If a patient refuses to make eye contact, you may find that they are _____.

   a. from a culture that considers direct eye contact rude.

   b. very tired.

   c. lying about their symptoms.

   d. disinterested in the conversation.

Section V – Insurance

1. What is the birthday rule?

   a. Methods to determine the primary insurance carrier when both parent's policy cover dependents.

   b. A method to determine the primary insurance carrier when both parents are covered.

   c. A method to determine the primary insurance carrier eligibility

   d. A method to determine the primary insurance carrier fees

2. What type of insurance generally covers workplace accidents?

   a. Medicare

   b. TRICARE

   c. Workers Compensation

   d. Patient's primary insurance carrier

3. What is an EOB?

   a. classification of diagnoses

   b. method to determine coverage

   c. a relative value unit

   d. a summary of services covered.

4. What is a method used by insurance carriers to determine prices based on prices charge by other carriers?

   a. Usual, Customary and Reasonable

   b. Reasonable Fee determination

   c. Usual Carrier Fees

   d. None of the Above

5. What is the process of determining how much or if the primary carrier will pay for a service?

    a. Predetermination

    b. Precertification

    c. Fee Quote

    d. None of the Above

6. What is the UCR fee of providers in an area called?

    a. Prevailing fee

    b. Customary fee

    c. Usual fee

    d. Local fee

7. What type of insurance carrier typically allows insured persons to select their own health care provider?

    a. Indemnity

    b. HMO

    c. Blue Cross

    d. TRICARE

8. What part of Medicare allows choice of a Medicare Advantage Plan?

    a. Part A

    b. Part B

    c. Part C

    d. Medicare does not allow choice of Medicare Advantage Plan

9. What is an Assignment of Benefits?

a. Authorization for the insurance company to send payments to the provider

b. Authorization for the insurance company to send payments to the insured person's spouse

c. Authorization for the insurance company to send payments to a deceased persons dependent

d. Authorization for the provider to perform the service

10. What is RVS?

a. The system for reimbursement

b. The relative values listed by procedure code

c. The component multiplied by a factor to calculate cost

d. None of the Above

11. What is Copayment?

a. Portion of total cost the insured person must pay

b. Portion of total cost paid by a spouses' insurance

c. Portion of total cost paid by the health care provider

d. Portion of total cost paid by the primary insurance carrier

12. What are diagnostic-related groups (DRG)?

a. Classification of diagnoses to determine hospital payment under Medicare

b. Classification of procedures to determine hospital payment under Medicare

c. Classification of diagnoses to determine hospital payment under TRICARE

d. Classification of diagnoses to determine insured payment under Medicare

13. What is Precertification?

a. Determining if a service is authorized.

b. Calculating the amount the carrier will pay for a service.

c. Obtaining approval for a service in advance.

d. Determining if a service is covered.

14. What is a third-party payer?

a. Whoever pays the doctor or hospital for the serviced given to the patient.

b. Whoever pays the patient for the services given by the doctor or hospital.

c. Whoever pays the primary carrier for the services provided to the patient.

d. None of the Above

Section VI – Records and Bookkeeping

15. What contains a listing of patients and amounts owing

a. Day sheet

b. General Ledger

c. Pegboard system

d. Account Receivable ledger

16. When a refund is made to a patient it is a(n)

a. Adjustment

b. Charge

c. Receivable

d. None of the Above

17. Monitoring overdue accounts is called

   a. reconciling
   b. auditing
   c. aging accounts
   d. checking

18. Accounts payable are considered a(n)

   a. asset
   b. liability
   c. neither asset nor liability

19. A customer check returned or bounced by the bank will be marked

   a. ISF
   b. NSF
   c. Bounced
   d. Returned

20. An endorsement is

   a. a signature on the front of a check
   b. a signature on the back of a check
   c. an initial on a check
   d. a signature on a contract

21. What is the tax withheld for Social Security and Medicare called?

   a. Social Security and Health Act (SSHA)
   b. Federal Insurance and Contribution Act (FICA)
   c. Federal Income tax
   d. Health and Security Act (HAS)

22. A purchase order

    a. is sent by the supplier to the medical office

    b. is sent by the medical office to a supplier

    c. is required by most insurance companies

    d. none of the above

23. The doctor has requested a discount for a patient. This is termed an

    a. account receivable

    b. account payable

    c. adjustment

    d. none of the above.

24. A check is not used or filled out in error. What should you do?

    a. Tear out and discard

    b. Mark Void

    c. Leave in check book

    d. None of the above

Section III – English and Spelling

1. Choose the sentence below with the correct punctuation.

a. Jessica's father was in the Navy, so she attended schools in Newark, New Jersey, Key West, Florida, San Diego, California, and Fairbanks, Alaska.

b. Jessica's father was in the Navy, so she attended schools in: Newark, New Jersey, Key West, Florida, San Diego, California, and Fairbanks, Alaska.

c. Jessica's father was in the Navy, so she attended schools in Newark, New Jersey; Key West, Florida; San Diego, California; and Fairbanks, Alaska.

d. Jessica's father was in the Navy, so she attended schools in Newark; New Jersey, Key West; Florida, San Diego, California, and Fairbanks, Alaska.

2. Choose the sentence below with the correct punctuation.

a. George wrecked John's car that was the end of their friendship.

b. George wrecked John's car. that was the end of their friendship.

c. George wrecked John's car; that was the end of their friendship.

d. None of the above

3. Choose the sentence below with the correct punctuation.

a. The dress was not Gina's favorite; however, she wore it to the dance.

b. The dress was not Gina's favorite, however, she wore it to the dance.

c. The dress was not Gina's favorite, however; she wore it to the dance.

d. The dress was not Gina's favorite however, she wore it to the dance.

4. Choose the sentence below with the correct punctuation.

a. Chris showed his dedication to golf in many ways, for example, he watched all of the tournaments on television.

b. Chris showed his dedication to golf in many ways; for example, he watched all of the   tournaments on television.

c. Chris showed his dedication to golf in many ways, for example; he watched all of the tournaments on television.

d. Chris showed his dedication to golf in many ways for example he watched all of the tournaments on television.

5. Choose the sentence with the correct grammar.

a. There was scarcely no food in the pantry, because nobody ate at home.

b. There was scarcely any food in the pantry, because nobody ate at home.

c. There was scarcely any food in the pantry, because not nobody ate at home.

d. There was scarcely no food in the pantry, because not nobody ate at home.

6. Choose the sentence with the correct grammar.

a. Although you may not see nobody in the dark, it does not mean that nobody is there.

b. Although you may not see anyone in the dark, it does not mean that not nobody is there.

c. Although you may not see anyone in the dark, it does not mean that anyone is there.

d. Although you may not see nobody in the dark, it does not mean that not nobody is there.

7. Choose the sentence with the correct grammar.

a. Michael has lived in that house for forty years, while I has owned this one for only six weeks.

b. Michael have lived in that house for forty years, while I have owned this one for only six weeks.

c. Michael have lived in that house for forty years, while I has owned this one for only six weeks.

d. Michael has lived in that house for forty years, while I have owned this one for only six weeks.

8. Choose the sentence with the correct grammar.

a. The older children have already eat their dinner, but the baby has not yet eaten anything.

b. The older children have already eaten their dinner, but the baby has not yet ate anything.

c. The older children have already eaten their dinner, but the baby has not yet eaten anything.

d. The older children have already eat their dinner, but the baby has not yet ate anything.

9. Choose the sentence with the correct grammar.

a. If they had gone to the party, he would have gone too.

b. If they had went to the party, he would have gone too.

c. If they had gone to the party, he would have went too.

d. If they had went to the party, he would have went too.

10. Choose the sentence with the correct grammar.

a. He should have went to the appointment; instead, he went to the beach.

b. He should have gone to the appointment; instead, he went to the beach.

c. He should have went to the appointment; instead, he gone to the beach.

d. He should have gone to the appointment; instead, he gone to the beach.

11. Choose the sentence with the correct grammar.

a. Lee pronounced it's name incorrectly; it's an i*mpatiens*, not an i*mpatience*.

b. Lee pronounced its name incorrectly; its an *impatiens*, not an *impatience*.

c. Lee pronounced it's name incorrectly; its an *impatiens*, not an *impatience*.

d. Lee pronounced its name incorrectly; it's an *impatiens*, not an *impatience*.

12. Choose the sentence with the correct grammar.

a. Its important for you to know its official name; its called the Confederate Museum.

b. It's important for you to know it's official name; it's called the Confederate Museum.

c. It's important for you to know its official name; it's called the Confederate Museum.

d. Its important for you to know it's official name; it's called the Confederate Museum.

13. The Ford Motor Company was named for Henry Ford _____.

    a. which had founded the company.

    b. who founded the company.

    c. whose had founded the company.

    d. whom had founded the company.

14. Thomas Edison _____ **after he invented the light bulb, television, motion pictures, and phonograph.**

    a. has always been known as the greatest inventor

    b. was always been known as the greatest inventor

    c. must have had been always known as the greatest inventor

    d. will had been known as the greatest inventor

15. The weatherman on Channel 6 said that this has been the _____.

    a. most hotter summer on record.

    b. most hottest summer on record.

    c. hottest summer on record.

    d. hotter summer on record.

16. Although Joe is tall for his age, his brother Elliot is _____ **of the two.**

    a. the tallest

    b. more tallest

    c. the tall

    d. the taller

17. I can never remember how to use those two common words, "sell," meaning to trade a product for money, or _____ meaning an event where products are traded for less money than usual.

    a. sale-

    b. "sale,"

    c. "sale

    d. "to sale,"

18. His father is _____.

    a. a poet and novelist

    b. poet and novelist

    c. a poet and a novelist

    d. None of the Above

19. The class just finished reading , _____ a short story by Carl Stephenson about a plantation owner's battle with army ants.

    a. -"Leinengen versus the Ants,"

    b. Leinengen versus the Ants,

    c. "Leinengen versus the Ants,"

    d. Leinengen versus the Ants

20. After the car was fixed it _____ again.

    a. ran good

    b. ran well

    c. would have run well

    d. ran more well

21. "Where does the sun go during the _____ asked little Kathy.

   a. night,"
   b. night?,"
   c. night,?"
   d. night?"

22. Choose the sentence with the correct usage.

   a. Vegetables are a healthy food; eating them can make you more healthful.

   b. Vegetables are a healthful food; eating them can make you more healthful.

   c. Vegetables are a healthy food; eating them can make you more healthy.

   d. Vegetables are a healthful food; eating them can make you more healthy.

23. Choose the sentence with the correct usage.

   a. When James went into his room, he found that his clothes had been put in the closet.

   b. When James went in his room, he found that his clothes had been put in the closet.

   c. When James went into his room, he found that his clothes had been put into the closet.

   d. When James went in his room, he found that his clothes had been put into the closet.

24. Choose the sentence with the correct usage.

a. After you lay the books on the counter, you may lay down for a nap.

b. After you lie the books on the counter, you may lay down for a nap.

c. After you lay the books on the counter, you may lie down for a nap.

d. After you lay the books on the counter, you may lay down for a nap.

25. Choose the sentence with the correct usage.

a. Once the chickens had layed their eggs, they lay on their nests to hatch them.

b. Once the chickens had lay their eggs, they lay on their nests to hatch them.

c. Once the chickens had laid their eggs, they lay on their nests to hatch them.

d. Once the chickens had laid their eggs, they laid on their nests to hatch them.

26. Choose the sentence with the correct usage.

a. Mrs. Foster taught me many things, but I learned the most from Mr. Wallace.

b. Mrs. Foster learned me many things, but I was taught the most by Mr. Wallace.

c. Mrs. Foster learned me many things, but I learned the most from Mr. Wallace.

d. Mrs. Foster taught me many things, but I was learned the most from Mr. Wallace.

27. Choose the sentence with the correct usage.

a. He did not have to loose the race; if only his shoes weren't so lose!

b. He did not have to lose the race; if only his shoes weren't so loose!

c. He did not have to loose the race; if only his shoes weren't so lose!

d. He did not have to loose the race; if only his shoes weren't so loose!

28. Choose the sentence with the correct usage.

a. The attorney did not want to prosecute the defendant; his goal was to prosecute the guilty party.

b. The attorney did not want to persecute the defendant; his goal was to persecute the guilty party.

c. The attorney did not want to prosecute the defendant; his goal was to persecute the guilty party.

d. The attorney did not want to persecute the defendant; his goal was to prosecute the guilty party.

29. Choose the sentence with the correct usage.

a. The speeches must precede the election; the election cannot proceed without hearing from the candidates.

b. The speeches must precede the election; the election cannot precede without hearing from the candidates.

c. The speeches must proceed the election; the election cannot precede without hearing from the candidates.

d. The speeches must proceed the election; the election cannot proceed without hearing from the candidates.

30. Choose the sentence with the correct capitalization.

   a. My best friend said, "always count your change."
   b. My best friend said, "Always Count your Change."
   c. My best friend said, "Always count your change."
   d. None of the above.

31. Choose the sentence with the correct capitalization.

   a. The Victorian Era was in the nineteenth century.
   b. The victorian era was in the nineteenth century.
   c. The Victorian Era was in the Nineteenth century.
   d. The Victorian era was in the Nineteenth century.

32. Choose the sentence with the correct capitalization.

   a. I prefer Pepsi to coke.
   b. I prefer pepsi to Coke.
   c. I prefer Pepsi to Coke.
   d. None of the above.

33. Choose the sentence with the correct capitalization.

   a. I always have french fries with my coke.
   b. I always have french fries with my Coke.
   c. I always have French Fries with my Coke.
   d. None of the above.

34. Choose the sentence with the correct capitalization.

   a. The blue jays are my favorite team.
   b. the blue Jays are my favorite team.
   c. The Blue Jays are my favorite team.
   d. None of the above.

35. Choose the sentence with the correct capitalization.

    a. The Southwest is the best part of the country.
    b. The southwest is the best part of the country.
    c. The southwest is the best part of the Country.
    d. None of the above.

Answer Key

Section I – Medical Terminology

1. A
Bodily organs can sometimes adhere to the **peritoneum**, a two-layered membrane lining the abdominal cavity and covering abdominal organs; when this occurs, it the problem is corrected through surgical release of **peritoneal adhesions**.

2. C
A/an **biopsy** allows a physician to obtain a small, representative sample of tissue for microscopic examination; this is usually done to establish a diagnosis.

3. A
Inguinal hernia repair is indicated when part of the intestine protrudes into the groin.

4. C
Hemorrhoids are distended veins in the lower rectum or anus; a **hemorrhoidectomy** is performed to relieve this condition.

5. B
During **open carpal tunnel surgery**, a tight band of transverse fibrous tissue is cut, releasing pressure on the median nerves and relieving symptoms.

6. A
A surgical procedure that unblocks the arteries located in the neck which supply blood to the brain is a/an **Carotid endarterectomy.**

7. D
Cataract surgery involves removal of the opaque contents of a lens of the eye via ultrasound waves, although, in some cases, the entire lens is removed and replaced with an artificial lens.

8. C
Following a radical hysterectomy, a small number of patients are placed on a hormone replacement regimen.

9. C
The following statement is false: **Fluoroscopy produces a series of still images of the body part being examined.**

Fluoroscopy is an imaging technique commonly used by physicians to obtain real-time moving images of the internal structures of a patient through the use of a fluoroscope. In its simplest form, a fluoroscope consists of an X-ray source and fluorescent screen between which a patient is placed. However, modern fluoroscopes couple the screen to an X-ray image intensifier and CCD video camera allowing the images to be recorded and played on a monitor.[38]

10. A
A/an **angiogram** is a test employed to identify blockages in the circulatory system, diagnose stroke and determine the size and location of brain tumors and aneurysms.

11. B
During a **biopsy**, a small sample of tissue is removed, usually under local anesthetic, examined microscopically for the purpose of diagnosis.

12. A
Electromyography (EMG) is a technique for evaluating and recording the electrical activity produced by skeletal muscles. EMG is performed using an instrument called an electromyograph, to produce a record called an electromyogram. An electromyograph detects the electrical potential generated by muscle cells when these cells are electrically or neurologically activated. The signals can be analyzed to detect medical abnormalities, activation level, and recruitment order or to analyze the biomechanics of human or animal movement.[39]

13. B
The following statement about cerebrospinal fluid analysis is false: **A lumbar puncture is performed to obtain a fluid sample, a painless procedure completed without the use**

of anesthetic.

CSF can be tested for the diagnosis of a variety of neurological diseases. It is usually obtained by a procedure called lumbar puncture. Removal of CSF during lumbar puncture can cause a severe headache after the fluid is removed, because the brain hangs on the vessels and nerve roots, and traction on them stimulates pain fibers. The pain can be relieved by intrathecal injection of sterile isotonic saline. Lumbar puncture is performed in an attempt to count the cells in the fluid and to detect the levels of protein and glucose. These parameters alone may be extremely beneficial in the diagnosis of subarachnoid hemorrhage and central nervous system infections (such as meningitis).[40]

14. D
Computed tomography, also known as a **CT scan**, is used to detect bone and vascular anomalies, certain types of brain tumors, and blood clots in patients who have experienced a stroke or brain damage due to an injury.

15. D
Using the magnetic properties of the blood, a **Functional MRI (fMRI)** produces real-time images of blood flow to certain areas of the brain and assesses damage due to head injury or disorders such as Alzheimer's disease.

16. C
The following statement is false, **PET scans are frequently used instead of CT or MRI scans, which are significantly less accurate.**

Note: Because they can provide additional information about specific areas of the brain, PET scans are sometimes ordered as a follow-up to the other tests.

Positron emission tomography (PET) is nuclear medicine imaging technique that produces a three-dimensional image or picture of functional processes in the body. The system detects pairs of gamma rays emitted indirectly by a positron-emitting radionuclide (tracer), which is introduced into the body on a biologically active molecule. The computer compiles three-dimensional images of tracer concentration in the body. In modern scanners, three-dimensional imaging is often accomplished with the aid of a CT X-ray scan performed on the patient during the same session, in the same machine.[41]

17. B
Physical medicine and rehabilitation (PM&R), physiatry or rehabilitation medicine, is a branch of medicine that aims to enhance and restore functional ability and quality of life to those with physical impairments or disabilities. A physician having completed training in this field is referred to as a physiatrist or rehab medicine specialist. Physiatrists specialize in restoring optimal function to people with injuries to the muscles, bones, tissues, and nervous system (such as stroke patients).[42]

18. D
Colorectal surgery is a field in medicine, dealing with disorders of the rectum, anus, and colon. The field is also known as proctology. Physicians specializing in this field of medicine are called colorectal surgeons or proctologists. [43]

19. D
Pulmonology (aka pneumology or respirology) is the specialty that deals with diseases of the respiratory tract and respiratory disease. It is called chest medicine and respiratory medicine in some countries and areas. Pulmonology is generally considered a branch of internal medicine, although it is closely related to intensive care medicine (aka critical care medicine) when dealing with patients requiring mechanical ventilation. Chest medicine is not a specialty in itself but is an inclusive term which pertains to the treatment of diseases of the chest and contains the fields of pulmonology, thoracic surgery, and intensive care medicine. [44]

20. B
Rheumatology is a sub-specialty in internal medicine and pediatrics, devoted to diagnosis and therapy of rheumatic diseases. Clinicians who specialize in rheumatology are called rheumatologists. Rheumatologists deal mainly with clinical problems involving joints, soft tissues, autoimmune diseases, vasculitis, and heritable connective tissue disorders.[45]

21. A
Vascular medicine, known in Europe as angiology, is a medical specialty centered on the study of the **circulatory** and **lymphatic** systems and diseases associated with those systems.

22. D
All for the statements are true.

> Thoracic surgeons treat diseases that affect the organs within the chest.
> Treatment most frequently involves conditions of the lungs, chest wall and diaphragm.
> Many times, thoracic surgery is grouped with cardiac surgery and termed cardiothoracic surgery.

23. B
Urology is the medical and surgical specialty that focuses on the urinary tracts of males and females, and on the reproductive system of males. Medical professionals specializing in the field of urology are called urologists and are trained to diagnose, treat, and manage patients with urological disorders. The organs covered by urology include the kidneys, adrenal glands, ureters, urinary bladder, urethra, and the male reproductive organs (testes, epididymis, vas deferens, seminal vesicles, prostate and penis). Urology is one of the most competitive specialties to enter for physicians.[46]

24. C
Cardiovascular surgery is surgery on the heart or great vessels performed by cardiac surgeons. Frequently, it is done to treat complications of ischemic heart disease (for example, coronary artery bypass grafting), correct congenital heart disease, or treat valvular heart disease from various causes including endocarditis, rheumatic heart disease and atherosclerosis. It also includes heart transplantation.[10]

25. D
The Greek prefix gastro-, in a medical context, means the stomach. For example, gastric bypass and gatronomy (art of good eating or putting healthy things in your stomach).

26. C
The Greek prefix gluco-, in a medical context, means sweet. For example, glucose and glucocorticoid.

27. B
The Greek prefix glyco-, in a medical context, means sugar.

28. C
The Latin prefix halluc-, in a medical context, meaningd wandering in mind. Examples are hallucinations and hallucinosis.

29. B
The Greek prefix hemi-, in a medical context, means one-half. For example the Cerebral hemisphere.

30. D
The Latin prefix huero- means the upper arm or shoulder. For example is humerus.
31. C
The Greek prefix hydro-, means water. For example, hydrophobia is the fear of water.

32. C
The Greek prefix hyper-, in a medical context, means something that is extreme or which is beyond normal. For example, hypertension is blood pressure which is higher than normal.

33. C
The Greek prefix hypo-, in a medical context, something that is below normal. For example, hypovolemia is a condition in which a person has a blood volume that is below normal.

34. B
The Latin prefix infra-, in a medical context, means below. For example, infrahyoid muscles are those below the hyoid muscles.

35. A
The Latin prefix intra- , in a medical context, means within. For example, an intracranial hemorrhage refers to blooding within the cranium.

36. B
The Greek prefix kerato-, in a medical context, means cornea, eye or skin. For example, a keratoscope is a device that helps to assess the shape of the surface of a person's cornea.

37. B
The Greek suffix -ac means pertaining to. An example in the medical context is cardiac, or pertaining to the heart.

38. C
The Greek suffix -acusis, , means of or for the sense of hearing. An example in a medical context is, paracusis or impaired hearing.

39. B
The Greek suffix -ase, means division. An example, in a medical context is lactase, or acts like a pair of molecule-scissors, dividing a lactose molecule into two parts.

40. D
The Greek suffix -cele, in a medical context, means pouching. An example is hydrocele, which refers to a collection of serous fluid in the body.

41. B
The Greek suffix, centesis, in a medical context, means a surgical puncture for aspiration. For example, amniocentesis.

42. D
The Latin suffix -cidal means destroying or killing. Examples are suicidal, which refers to someone intent on taking his own life, or homicidal, designating someone who has a tendency to kill or want to kill others.

43. A
The Greek suffix -desis means binding. An example in a medical context, is arthrodesis, which is the surgical binding of a patient's joint where there is pain; the procedure is done to release the pressure causing the pain.

44. A
The suffix -dynia, often used in a medical context, means pain. An example is vulvodynia, chronic pain around the vulvar area.

45. B
The Greek suffix -ectomy, in a medical context, means surgery to remove either a body part or a portion of a body part. For example, an appedectomy is a procedure to take out the appendix, while a tonsillectomy is to remove one's tonsils.

46. A
The Greek suffix -emia, in a medical context, refers to: a. a condition of the blood. A classic exammple is anemia, which refers to having too few blood cells.

47. C
The Greek suffix -ist, means one who specializes. For example, in a medical context, a cardiologist specializes in the heart, while a podiatrist specializes in the feet.

48. D
The suffix -itis, in a medical context, means inflammation. For example, tonsillitis is an inflammation of the tonsils.

49. D
The Greek suffix -lepsy, in a medical context, means an attack or seizure. For example, epilepsy is a condition that causes many seizures.

50. A
The Greek suffix -logy means study. For example, biology is the study of life, and urology is the study of urinary conditions.

51. B
The Greek suffix -meter means something used to count or measure. For example, a thermometer measures the body temperature.

52. C
The Greek suffix -oid means resembling something else.

For example, sarcoidosis literally means 'flesh-like diseased condition.'

53. D
The Greek suffix -oma or -omata, in a medical context, means a mass or tumor. For example, sarcoma is a malignant tumor made of fat, cartilage, bone, muscle, and hematopoietic or vascular tissues.

54. B
The Greek suffix -osis, used often in a medical context means a condition. For example, osteoperosis is a deterioration of the bones.

55. A
The Greek suffix -pathy, in a medical context, means a disease or disorder. For example, neuropathy refers to a disease or disorder that creates damage to the nerves within the peripheral nervous system.

56. D
The Greek suffix -plasty, used often in a medical context, means reconstruction or surgical repair. For example, rhinoplasty refers to a surgical reconstruction of the nose.

57. B
The Greek suffix -rrhage means bursting forth. For example, a hemorrhage is a sudden, violent bleeding within the body.

58. C
The Latin suffix, -tension, in a medical context, means pressure. For example, hypertension refers to high blood pressure.

59. A
AED stands for Automated External Defibrillator. This is the machine used to revive the heart after it has gone into full arrest.

60. B
A.C. stands for before meals. This is used most often on prescriptions, telling the patient when to take the medication.

Practice Test Questions Set 2 187

Section II – Anatomy and Physiology

1. D
Osteoporosis is a disease of bones that leads to an increased risk of fracture. In osteoporosis the bone mineral density (BMD) is reduced, bone micro-architecture is deteriorating, and the amount and variety of proteins in bone is altered. The disease may be classified as primary type 1, primary type 2, or secondary [47]

2. D
Marfan syndrome (also called Marfan's syndrome) is a genetic disorder of the connective tissue. People with Marfan's tend to be unusually tall, with long limbs and long, thin fingers. [48]

3. D
The **circulatory system** can be thought of as the blood distribution system.

4. B
The circulatory system is an organ system that passes nutrients (such as amino acids, electrolytes and lymph), gases, hormones, blood cells, etc. to and from cells in the body to help fight diseases and help stabilize body temperature and pH to maintain homeostasis.[49]

5. C
The circulatory system is an organ system that passes nutrients (such as amino acids, electrolytes and lymph), gases, hormones, blood cells, etc. to and from cells in the body to help fight diseases and help stabilize body temperature and pH to maintain homeostasis. [49]

6. A
The main components of the circulatory system are the heart, veins and blood vessels.

7. D
The circulatory system disease that is one of the most frequent causes of death in North America is **heart disease**.

8. C
Angina is frequently mistaken for a heart attack. Angina

pectoris, commonly known as angina, is severe chest pain due to ischemia (a lack of blood, thus a lack of oxygen supply) of the heart muscle, generally due to obstruction or spasm of the coronary arteries (the heart's blood vessels).[50]

9. B
High blood pressure is a more common name for the circulatory system disease known as hypertension. Hypertension (HTN) or high blood pressure is a cardiac chronic medical condition in which the systemic arterial blood pressure is elevated.

10. D
Cardiac dysrhythmia (also known as arrhythmia and irregular heartbeat) is a term for any of a large and heterogeneous group of conditions in which there is abnormal electrical activity in the heart. The heartbeat may be too fast or too slow, and may be regular or irregular.[51]

11. A
The respiratory system is the anatomical system of an organism that introduces respiratory gases to the interior and performs gas exchange. The anatomical features of the respiratory system include airways, lungs, and the respiratory muscles. Molecules of oxygen and carbon dioxide are passively exchanged, by diffusion, between the gaseous external environment and the blood. This exchange process occurs in the alveolar region of the lungs [52]

12. B
The Lungs are an important component of the respiratory system.

13. D
The exchange of oxygen for carbon dioxide takes place in the alveolar area of **the lungs**.

14. B
The thoracic diaphragm, or simply the diaphragm, is a sheet of internal skeletal muscle that extends across the bottom of the rib cage. The diaphragm separates the thoracic cavity (heart, lungs & ribs) from the abdominal cavity and **performs an important function in respiration**.[53]

15. A
Exhalation is often accomplished by the **abdominal muscles**.

16. D
The blood is the primary thing oxygenated through the work of the respiratory system.

17. C
An important side-benefit of the respiratory system is the air being expelled from the mouth allows for speaking.

18. A
Emphysema is a long-term, progressive disease of the lungs that primarily causes shortness of breath. In people with emphysema, the tissues necessary to support the physical shape and function of the lungs are destroyed. It is included in a group of diseases called chronic obstructive pulmonary disease or COPD (pulmonary refers to the lungs).[54]

19. C
The immune system is **the system that protects the body from disease and infection.**

20. A
The immune system fights off disease by **identifying and killing tumor cells and pathogens.**

21. D
An example of a pathogen that the immune system detects is **A virus**.

22. A
Detection of pathogens can be complicated because **they evolve so quickly.**

23. B
One of the best-known disorders that attack the immune system is **HIV (the virus that causes AIDS).**

24. A
The process by which the immune system adapts over time to be more efficient in recognizing pathogens is known as

acquired immunity.

25. B
Inflammation is an example of an early response by the immune system to infection.

26. B
White blood cells are an important weapon in the fight against infection.

27. D
The primary purpose of the digestive system is **to convert food into a form that can provide nourishment for the body.**

28. A
Gastric acid is a digestive fluid, formed in the stomach. It has a pH of 1 to 2 and is composed of hydrochloric acid (HCl) (around 0.5%, or 5000 parts per million), and large quantities of potassium chloride (KCl) and sodium chloride (NaCl). The acid plays a key role in digestion of proteins, by activating digestive enzymes, and making ingested proteins unravel so that digestive enzymes can break down the long chains of amino acids.[55]

29. D
Digestion begins **in the mouth.**

30. B
Cleansing food of impurities is not an example of a function of the stomach in digestion.

31. A
Fats stay in the stomach longest.

32. C
Indigestion is a common digestive affliction that most people suffer at one time or other.

33. B
Diverticulitis is a pouch in the large intestine becomes inflamed.

34. A
Eating a healthy diet is the best way to avoid most digestive diseases.

35. D
Producing, storing and eliminating urine are the three functions of the urinary system.

36. B
Urine **is mostly comprised of waste material after the body has taken the nutrients from food and absorbed the water it needs.**

37. A
Urea is the name of the waste removed from the body through urine.

38. B
Carrying urea to the kidneys is one example of the blood stream's part in the digestive system.

39. D
Besides the kidney, the other major organ that takes part in the body's urinary system is **the Bladder**

40. B
The bladder **is a balloon shaped, muscular organ.**

41. C
Kidney failure is an example of one of the many serious urinary disorders.

42. A
The involuntary passage of urine defines the urinary-system disorder known as **incontinence**.

43. A
The lymphatic system is the system which **carries a clear liquid lymph toward the heart.**

44. B
Lymphoid tissue **exists in many organs, although it's predominantly in the lymph nodes.**

45. C
An example of an organ that plays a big role in the lymphatic system is **the spleen.**

46. D
Among the benefits of the lymphatic system is the fact that it **Absorbs and transports fats and fatty acids from the body's circulatory system.**

47. A
Metastasis is a **process of carrying cancer cells between various parts of the body.**

48. B
A common affliction of the lymphatic system is **swelling of the lymph nodes**.

49. A
An example of a cause of lymph node swelling is **Infectious mononucleosis ("Mono").**

50. D
Another, more serious, example of a cause of lymph node swelling is **cancer.**

Section III – Medical Law, Ethics and Legislation

1. C
In many U.S. states and Australia, **mandated reporters** are professionals who, in the ordinary course of their work and because they have regular contact with children, disabled persons, senior citizens, or other identified vulnerable populations, are required to report (or cause a report to be made) whenever financial, physical, sexual or other types of abuse has been observed or is suspected, or when there is evidence of neglect, knowledge of an incident, or an imminent risk of serious harm. For example, in South Australia, a school teacher must report a child attending school seeming malnourished or presenting with bruising, complaining of neglect or otherwise demonstrating neglect or abuse at home, to child welfare authorities.

These professionals can be held liable by both the civil and criminal legal systems for intentionally failing to make a report but their name can also be said unidentified. Mandated reporters also include persons who have assumed full or intermittent responsibility for the care or custody of a child, dependent adult, or elder, whether or not they are compensated for their services. RAINN maintains a database of mandatory reporting regulations regarding children and the elderly by state, including who is required to report, standards of knowledge, definitions of a victim, to whom the report must be made, information required in the report, and regulations regarding timing and other procedures.[56]

2. A
Signs of physical child abuse may include but are not limited to:

- Inability to recall how injuries occurred or offers an inconsistent explanation
- wary of adults
- may cringe or flinch if touched unexpectedly
- infants may display a vacant stare
- extremely aggressive or extremely withdrawn
- indiscriminately seeks affection
- extremely compliant and/or eager to please

3. A
Signs of emotional abuse may include but are not limited to:

- severe depression
- Non-attachment to the parent
- extreme withdrawal or aggressiveness
- overly compliant, too well mannered, too neat or clean
- extreme attention seeking
- displays extreme inhibition in play

4. D
Signs of sexual abuse may include but are not limited to:

- age inappropriate play with toys, self or others displaying explicit sexual acts
- age inappropriate sexually explicit drawing and/or

descriptions
- bizarre, sophisticated or unusual sexual knowledge
- prostitution
- seductive behaviors

5. D
Child neglect is defined as:

- "the failure of a person responsible for a child's care and upbringing to safeguard the child's emotional and physical health and general well-being"
- acts of commission, harm to a child may or may not be the intended consequence
- a serious form of maltreatment
- the persistent failure to meet a child's basic physical and/or psychological needs resulting in serious impairment of health and/or development.[57]

6. D
All of the following are signs of fetal abuse:

- Poor fetal growth on abdomen measurements or ultrasound
- History or signs of domestic abuse
- History or signs of maternal alcohol or drug use

7. D
The following statements are used by the Uniform Determination of Death Act (UDDA) to define death

- The individual has sustained irreversible cessation of circulatory and respiratory functions.
- The individual has sustained irreversible cessation of all functions of the entire brain, including the brain stem.

8. B
Malfeasance is also known as misfeasance and nonfeasance.

9. C
Government agencies such as Medicare, Workers Compensation and Social Security Disability Insurance

10. A
The medical information of a person at risk for HIV being released without patient permission in an emergency situation to medical personnel or a court order has been issued.

.11. B
Distributive justice refers to what society owes a person in proportion to their individual needs and responsibilities, the resources available and society's responsibilities to the common good.

12. A
The term managed care is used in the United States to describe a variety of techniques intended to reduce the cost of providing health benefits and improve the quality of care ("managed care techniques") for organizations that use those techniques or provide them as services to other organizations ("managed care organization" or "MCO"), or to describe systems of financing and delivering health care to enrollees organized around managed care techniques and concepts ("managed care delivery systems"). According to the United States National Library of Medicine, the term "managed care" encompasses programs:

...intended to reduce unnecessary health care costs through a variety of mechanisms, including: economic incentives for physicians and patients to select less costly forms of care; programs for reviewing the medical necessity of specific services; increased beneficiary cost sharing; controls on inpatient admissions and lengths of stay; the establishment of cost-sharing incentives for outpatient surgery; selective contracting with health care providers; and the intensive management of high-cost health care cases. The programs may be provided in a variety of settings, such as Health Maintenance Organizations and Preferred Provider Organizations.[58]

13. B
Benefits available to immigrants include school lunch and breakfast programs, immunizations, emergency medical services, disaster relief, and others programs that are necessary to protect life and safety as identified by the

attorney general, regardless of immigration status

14. C
A **Do Not Resuscitate (DNR)** indicates that a patient does not want cardiopulmonary resuscitation or defibrillation at the end of life, while a **DNI order** indicates that the patient rejects the use of a breathing tube in cases of respiratory arrest. **Both** can be revoked at any time.

A "do not resuscitate" or "DNR" , sometimes called a "No Code," is a legal order written either in the hospital or on a legal form to respect the wishes of a patient to not undergo CPR or advanced cardiac life support (ACLS) if their heart were to stop or they were to stop breathing. The term "code" is commonly used by medical professionals as a slang term for "calling in a Code Blue" to alert a hospital's resuscitation team. This request is usually made by the patient or health care power of attorney and allows the medical teams taking care of them to respect their wishes. In the health care community "allow natural death" or "AND" is a term that is quickly gaining favor as it focuses on what is being done, not what is being avoided. Some criticize the term "do not resuscitate" because it sounds as if something important is being withheld, while research shows that only about 5% of patients who require ACLS outside the hospital and only 15% of patients who require ACLS while in the hospital survive. Elderly patients living in nursing homes have multiple medical problems, or who have advanced cancer are much less likely to survive.[59]

15. C
In American law, competence concerns the mental capacity of an individual to participate in legal proceedings. Defendants that do not possess sufficient "competence" are usually excluded from criminal prosecution, while witnesses found not to possess requisite competence cannot testify. The English equivalent is fitness to plead. [60]

16. B
Civil law, as opposed to criminal law, is the branch of law dealing with disputes between individuals or organizations, in which compensation may be awarded to the victim. For instance, if a car crash victim claims damages against the

driver for loss or injury sustained in an accident, this will be a civil law case.

Civil law is usually referred to in comparison to criminal law, which is that body of law involving the state against individuals (including incorporated organizations) where the state relies on the power given it by statutory law. [61]

17. D
Cultural competence refers to an ability to interact effectively with people of different **cultures**.

Cultural competence refers to an ability to interact effectively with people of different cultures, particularly in the context of human resources, non-profit organizations, and government agencies whose employees work with persons from different cultural/ethnic backgrounds.
Cultural competence comprises four components: (a) Awareness of one's own cultural worldview, (b) Attitude towards cultural differences, (c) Knowledge of different cultural practices and worldviews, and (d) cross-cultural skills. Developing cultural competence results in an ability to understand, communicate with, and effectively interact with people across cultures.[60]

18. A
A 2006 follow-up to the 2000 Institute of Medicine study found that medication errors are among the most common medical mistakes, harming at least 1.5 million people every year. According to the study, 400,000 preventable drug-related injuries occur each year in hospitals, 800,000 in long-term care settings, and roughly 530,000 among Medicare recipients in outpatient clinics. The report stated that these are likely to be conservative estimates. In 2000 alone, the extra medical costs incurred by preventable drug related injuries approximated $887 million — and the study looked only at injuries sustained by Medicare recipients, a subset of clinic visitors. None of these figures take into account lost wages and productivity or other costs.

According to a 2002 Agency for Healthcare Research and Quality report, about 7,000 people were estimated to die each year from medication errors - about 16 percent more deaths than the number attributable to work-related injuries (6,000 deaths)[62]

19. D
Types of medication errors include:

- Administration errors which occur when the provider gives the wrong medicine to the patient
- Pharmacy fulfillment errors
- Transcription errors which occur when the pharmacist misreads the prescription or it is written incorrectly

20. A
The law demands that patients are treated compassionately, while ethics require competent medical practice according to current standards and frequently exceed legal standards.

21. D
A medical professional cannot refuse to treat a patient with an infectious disease.

22. C
The Health Insurance Portability and Accountability Act of 1996 was enacted by the U.S. Congress and signed by President Bill Clinton in 1996.

Title I of HIPAA protects health insurance coverage for workers and their families when they change or lose their jobs.

Title II of HIPAA, known as the Administrative Simplification (AS) provisions, requires the establishment of national standards for electronic health care transactions and national identifiers for providers, health insurance plans, and employers.

The Administration Simplification provisions also address the security and privacy of health data. The standards are meant to improve the efficiency and effectiveness of the nation's health care system by encouraging the widespread use of electronic data interchange in the U.S. health care system. [63]

23. C
Adolescents must always obtain parental permission before placing a child for adoption.

24. A
An **emancipated minor** is a minor who is allowed to conduct a business or any other occupation on his or her own behalf or for their own account outside the influence of a parent or guardian. The minor will then have full contractual capacity to conclude contract with regard to the business. Whether parental consent is needed to achieve the "emancipated" status varies from case to case. In some cases, court permission is necessary. Protocols vary by jurisdiction. [64]

25. A
A fiduciary duty is a legal or ethical relationship of confidence or trust between two or more parties. Typically, a fiduciary prudently takes care of money for another person.

26. D
The United States Department of Health and Human Services oversees the FDA. Formerly, this department was known simply as the Department of Health.

27. C
The FDA is responsible for promoting health through regulating and supervising food safety, dietary supplements, pharmaceutical drugs and **tobacco**. Clothing does not come under their oversight because it is not consumed by humans. The same applies to livestock feeMarijuana is not in their jurisdiction since they oversee prescription (legal) medications.[65]

28. B
Laundry detergent is not regulated by the FDA. Non-edible and non-medical products on sale at the retail level are generally under the oversight of the Consumer Protection Agency.

29. C
The Commissioner of Food & Drugs leads the FDA. This official is appointed by the President of the United States

and must be approved by the U.S. Senate.

30. B
ADA, when referring to the 1990s law that covers Americans with disabilities, stands for Americans with Disabilities Act.

Section IV – Communication Skills and Patient Education

1. B
Level of education can act as a barrier to communication.

2. A
Personal space is the zone around each person reserved for **conversation** and can vary according to **culture.**

3. D
When dealing with elderly patients, always **address them as Miss, Mrs., or Mr., followed by their last name.**

4. B
A complete medical history should include **the chief complaint.**

5. C
When documenting a patient's chief complaint, be careful to **use the patient's exact words.**

6. D
Physical barriers to communication include**, time, environment, and
Illness.**

7. A
If a patient does not seem to understand a question, **repeat the question using simpler terms.** Asking if they understand or skipping the question are not helpful.

8. D
Perception checking is repeating what someone has said to check the accuracy of the information.

9. C
For patients who are depressed, cognitively impaired, or unable to deal with complex communication at that particular moment, using **direct questions** that require short answers can help obtain information.

10. B
Silence should always be avoided in the interview process is false. Silence can be very useful during an interview, as it can allow patients to think about their answer.

11. C
A leading question is a question that suggests the answer.

12. A
Leading questions are an ineffective means of obtaining information because **the patient may feel forced to give the answer the interviewer is looking for.**

13. D
During the interview process, the most accurate information is provided by **the patient.**

14. A
When interviewing a patient with a hearing loss, remember to Speak slowly and look directly at the patient.

15. D
The medical record is the key means of communication between healthcare workers.

16. B
A **health history** is used to obtain **subjective** information and learn about past and current health problems.

17. C
Biographic information is the first area to be covered when obtaining a health history.

18. C
Using neutral remarks such as, "I see" and "I hear what you're saying" indicates **understanding** to the patient.

19. D
In addition to providing **accurate** patient information to other healthcare professionals, it is necessary that one be able to **interpret** what others have added to the medical record.

20. A
If a patient refuses to make eye contact, you may find that they are **from a culture that considers direct eye contact rude.**

Section V – Insurance

1. B
The Birthday Rule is where a person is covered by two insurance policies. The policy to be billed is determined by the policyholder whose birthday comes first in the calendar year.

2. C
Workers' Compensation is a form of insurance providing wage replacement and medical benefits to employees injured in the course of employment in exchange for mandatory relinquishment of the employee's right to sue his or her employer for the tort of negligence. The trade-off between assured, limited coverage and lack of recourse outside the worker compensation system is known as "the compensation bargain."

3. D
AN EOB, also called remittance advice, is an explanation of what is covered and what is not covered and why.

4. A
Some insurance companies use a method called, Usual, Customary and Reasonable that compares Physician's charges for a procedure in a geographical area.

5. B
Precertification, also knows as preauthorization. Most insurance companies require precertification 24 hours before a patient is admitted or undergoes certain procedures.

6. A
Usual, Customary and Reasonable is also called the Prevailing Fee.

7. A
An Indemnity Plan is a health insurance plan where all or a part of the costs are covered, for any physician, hospital or licensed provider.

8. C
Starting in 1997, Medicare beneficiaries were given the option to receive their Medicare benefits through private health insurance plans, instead of through the original Medicare plan (Parts A and B). These programs were known as "Medicare+Choice" or "Part C" plans.

"Medicare+Choice" plans were made more attractive to Medicare beneficiaries by the addition of prescription drug coverage and became known as "Medicare Advantage" (MA) plans. Medicare Advantage plans are offered through private companies known as Medicare Advantage Organizations (MAO). Each of them under the contract from CMS are required to provide an effective compliance program to prevent Fraud, Waste and Abuse issues in healthcare settings.

9. A
Assignment of benefits authorizes payment to be sent to the provider. In fact, the assignment of benefits is the transfer of the patient's legal right to collect benefits to the provider.

10. B
Relative Value Studies list the procedure codes and relative values, allowing a comparison of costs for the different codes.

11. A
Copayment, also called coinsurance, is the cost or percentage the insured person pays.

12. A
Diagnosis-related group (DRG) is a system to classify hospital cases into one of originally 467 groups. The 467th was "Ungroupable." The system is also referred to as

"the DRGs," and its intent was to identify the "products" that a hospital provides. One example of a "product" is an appendectomy. The system was developed at Yale, in anticipation of convincing Congress to use it for reimbursement, to replace "cost based" reimbursement that was used up to that point. DRGs are assigned by a "grouper" program based on ICD (International Classification of Diseases) diagnoses, procedures, age, sex, discharge status, and the presence of complications or comorbidities. DRGs have been used in the US since 1982 to determine how much Medicare pays the hospital for each "product," since patients within each category are similar clinically and are expected to use the same level of hospital resources. DRGs may be further grouped into Major Diagnostic Categories (MDCs).[66]

13. D
Precertification, also knows as preauthorization. Most insurance companies require precertification 24 hours before a patient is admitted or undergoes certain procedures.

14. A
A Third-Party Payer is who ever pays the doctor or hospital for services, usually a public or private insurance company.

Section VI – Records and Bookkeeping

15. D
Accounts receivable represents money owed by entities to the firm on the sale of products or services on credit. In most business entities, accounts receivable is typically executed by generating an invoice and either mailing or electronically delivering it to the customer, who, in turn, must pay it within an established timeframe, called credit terms or payment terms.[67]

16. A
An adjustment in accounting is a change to the amount owed for reasons other than payments or changes in services, such as a refund or discount.

17. C
Accounts Receivable accounts are monitored with the Accounts Receivable Age Analysis Printout, also known as the Debtors Book is divided in categories for current, 30 days, 60 days, 90 days, 120 days, 150 days and 180 days and over due that are produced in Modern Accounting Systems. The printout is done in the order of the Chart of Accounts for the Accounts Receivable and/or Debtors Book.[67]

18. B
Accounts payable are a Liability for the business.

19. B
A customer check returned by the bank will be marked NSF for Not Sufficient Funds.

20. B
To endorse a check is to sign the back.

21. B
Tax withheld for Social Security and Medicare is called the Federal Insurance and Contribution Act (FICA).

22. B
A purchase order is sent to the supplier by the medical office.

23. C
An adjustment in accounting is a change to the amount owed for reasons other than payments or changes in services, such as a refund or discount.

24. B
Checks that you aren't going to use should be marked Void to prevent use by unauthorized persons.

Section VII – Fundamental Writing Skills

1. C
The semicolon is used in a list where the list items have internal punctuation, such as "Key West, Florida."

2. C
The semicolon links independent clauses.

3. A
The semicolon links independent clauses with a conjunction (However).

4. B
The semicolon links independent clauses.

5. B
Double negative sentence. In double negative sentences, one of the negatives is replaced with "any."

6. C
Double negative sentence. In double negative sentences, one of the negatives is replaced with "any."

7. D
Present perfect. You cannot use the Present Perfect with specific time expressions such as: yesterday, one year ago, last week, when I was a child, at that moment, that day, one day, etc. The Present Perfect is used with unspecific expressions such as: ever, never, once, many times, several times, before, so far, already, yet, etc.

8. C
Present perfect. You cannot use the Present Perfect with specific time expressions such as: yesterday, one year ago, last week, when I was a child, at that moment, that day, one day, etc. The Present Perfect is used with unspecific expressions such as: ever, never, once, many times, several times, before, so far, already, yet, etc.

9. A
Went vs. Gone. Went is the simple past tense. Gone is used in the past perfect.

10. B
Went vs. Gone. Went is the simple past tense. Gone is used in the past perfect.

11. D
Its vs. It's. It's is a contraction for it is or it has. Its is a possessive pronoun meaning, more or less, of it or belonging to it.

12. C
Its vs. It's. It's is a contraction for it is or it has. Its is a possessive pronoun meaning, more or less, of it or belonging to it.

13. B
"Who" is the best option because the sentence refers to a person.

14. A
The sentence is past perfect.

15. C
The superlative "hottest" is used when expressing the highest degree, or a degree greater than that of anything it is being compared with.

16. C
When comparing 2, use "the taller." When comparing more than 2, use the tallest.

17. B

18. C

19. C
Titles of short stories are enclosed in quotation marks, and commas always go inside quotation marks.

20. B
Present tense, "ran well" is correct. "Ran good" is never correct.

21. D
Punctuation always goes inside quotation marks.

22. D
Healthful vs. Healthy. Healthy should be used to describe something that is of good for your health and Healthful refers to habits or types.

23. A
In vs. Into. In a room means inside. Into refers to movement or action.

24. C
Lay vs. Lie. Lie requires an object and lay does not. So you can lie down, (no object. and you lay a book on the floor.

25. C
Lay vs. Lie. Lie requires an object and lay does not. Laid is the past tense of lay .

26. B
Learn vs. Teach. Learning is what students do, and teaching is what teachers do.

27. B
Lose vs. Loose. Lose is to no longer have, or to lose a race. Loose is not tied or able to move freely.

28. D
Persecute vs. Prosecute. To prosecute is to have a legal claim against someone and to persecute is to harass.

29. A
Precede vs. Proceed. To precede is to go first or in front of. To proceed is to go forward.

30. C
Quoted speech is not capitalized.

31. A
Periods and events are capitalized but not century numbers.

32. C
Brand names are capitalized.

33. B
Brand names are capitalized by generic terms such as 'french fries' are not.

34. C
The names of sports teams, as proper nouns, are capitalized.

35. A
North, South, East, and West when used as sections of the country, but not as compass directions

Conclusion

CONGRATULATIONS! You have made it this far because you have applied yourself diligently to practicing for the exam and no doubt improved your potential score considerably! Getting into a good school is a huge step in a journey that might be challenging at times but will be many times more rewarding and fulfilling. That is why being prepared is so important.

Study then Practice and then Succeed!

Good Luck!

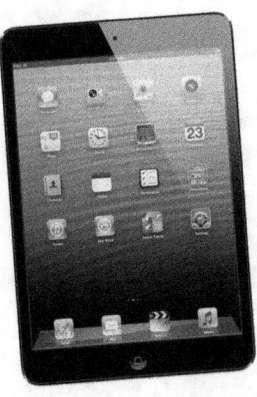

FREE Ebook Version

Download a FREE Ebook version of the publication!

Suitable for tablets, iPad, iPhone, or any smart phone.

Go to
http://tinyurl.com/

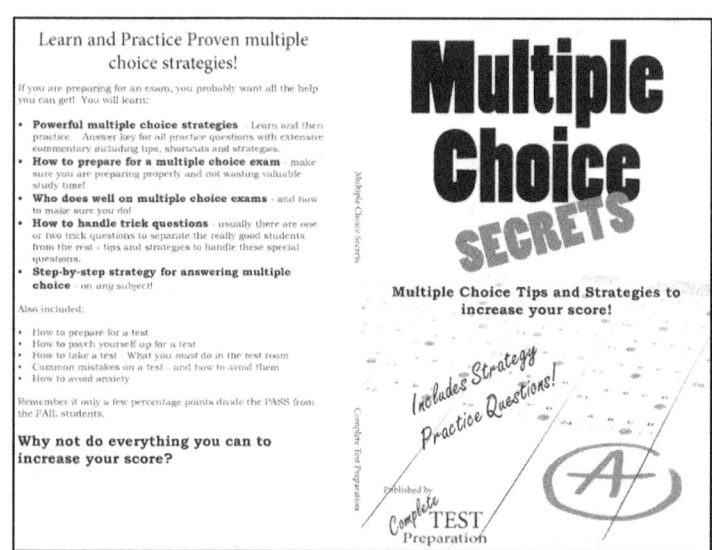

Multiple Choice Secrets!

Learn to increase your score using time-tested secrets for answering multiple choice questions!

This practice book has everything you need to know about answering multiple choice questions on a standardized test!

You will learn 12 strategies for answering multiple choice questions and then practice each strategy with over 45 reading comprehension multiple choice questions, with extensive commentary from exam experts!

Maybe you have read this kind of thing before, and maybe feel you don't need it, and you are not sure if you are going to buy this Book.

Even if our multiple choice strategies increase your score by a few percentage points, isn't that worth it?

Go to www.multiple-choice.ca start learning multiple choice secrets!

Notes

[1] Geriatrician. In Wikipedia. Retrieved November 12, 2010 from http://en.wikipedia.org/wiki/Geriatrician
[2] Palliative Medicine. In Wikipedia. Retrieved November 12, 2010 from http://en.wikipedia.org/wiki/Palliative_medicine.
[3] Nephrology. In Wikipedia. Retrieved November 12, 2010 from http://en.wikipedia.org/wiki/Nephrologists.
[4] Oncology. In Wikipedia. Retrieved November 12, 2010 from http://en.wikipedia.org/wiki/Oncology.
[5] Pathology. In Wikipedia. Retrieved November 12, 2010 from http://en.wikipedia.org/wiki/Pathology.
[6] Homeostasis. In Wikipedia. Retrieved November 12, 2010 from http://en.wikipedia.org/wiki/Human_homeostasis.
[7] Cell Membrane. In Wikipedia. Retrieved November 12, 2010 from http://en.wikipedia.org/wiki/Cell_membrane.
[8] Mitosis. In *Wikipedia*. Retrieved November 12, 2010 from http://en.wikipedia.org/wiki/Mitosis.
[9] Prophase. In *Wikipedia*. Retrieved November 12, 2010 from http://en.wikipedia.org/wiki/Prophase.
[10] Metaphase. In *Wikipedia*. Retrieved November 12, 2010 from http://en.wikipedia.org/wiki/Metaphase.
[11] Anaphase. In *Wikipedia*. Retrieved November 12, 2010 from http://en.wikipedia.org/wiki/Anaphase.
[12] Telophase. In *Wikipedia*. Retrieved November 12, 2010 from http://en.wikipedia.org/wiki/Telophase.
[13] In *Wikipedia*. Retrieved November 12, 2010 from http://en.wikipedia.org/wiki/Epithelial_tissue.
[14] Integumentary. In Wikipedia. Retrieved November 12, 2010 from http://en.wikipedia.org/wiki/Integumentary.
[15] Cartilage. In Wikipedia. Retrieved November 12, 2010 from http://en.wikipedia.org/wiki/Cartilage.

[17] Battery. In Wikipedia. Retrieved November 12, 2010 from http://en.wikipedia.org/wiki/Battery_(crime).
[18] Medical Ethics. In Wikipedia. Retrieved November 12, 2010 from http://en.wikipedia.org/wiki/Medical_ethics.
[19] Double Effect. http://en.wikipedia.org/wiki/Double_effect
[20] Beneficence. http://en.wikipedia.org/wiki/Beneficence_(ethics)#Beneficence
[21] Triage. In Wikipedia. Retrieved November 12, 2010 from

http://en.wikipedia.org/wiki/Triage.
[22] Informed Consent. In Wikipedia. Retrieved November 12, 2010 from http://en.wikipedia.org/wiki/Informed_consent.
[23] Medical Malpractice. In Wikipedia. Retrieved November 12, 2010 from http://en.wikipedia.org/wiki/Medical_malpractice.
[24] Tort Law. In Wikipedia. Retrieved November 12, 2010 from http://en.wikipedia.org/wiki/Tort_law
[25] Advance Directive. In Wikipedia. Retrieved November 12, 2010 from http://en.wikipedia.org/wiki/Advance_directive.
[26] Uniform Anatomical Gift Act. In Wikipedia. Retrieved November 12, 2010 from http://en.wikipedia.org/wiki/Uniform_Anatomical_Gift_Act.
[27] Health Maintenance Organization. In Wikipedia. Retrieved November 12, 2010 from http://en.wikipedia.org/wiki/Health_maintenance_organization.
[28] Preferred Provider Organization. In Wikipedia. Retrieved November 12, 2010 from http://en.wikipedia.org/wiki/Preferred_provider_organization.
[29] Tricare. In Wikipedia. Retrieved November 12, 2010 from http://en.wikipedia.org/wiki/Tricare.
[30] Medicare US. In Wikipedia. Retrieved November 12, 2010 from http://en.wikipedia.org/wiki/Medicare_(United_States).
[31] Relative Value Units. In Wikipedia. Retrieved November 12, 2010 from http://en.wikipedia.org/wiki/Relative_Value_Units.
[32] Workers Compensation. In Wikipedia. Retrieved November 12, 2010 from http://en.wikipedia.org/wiki/Workers_compensation.
[33] RBRVS. In Wikipedia. Retrieved November 12, 2010 from http://en.wikipedia.org/wiki/RBRVS.
[34] Petty Cash. In Wikipedia. Retrieved November 12, 2010 from http://en.wikipedia.org/wiki/Petty_cash.
[35] Accounts Payable. In Wikipedia. Retrieved November 12, 2010 from http://en.wikipedia.org/wiki/Accounts_payable.
[36] Bill of Lading. In Wikipedia. Retrieved November 12, 2010 from http://en.wikipedia.org/wiki/Bill_of_lading.
[37] Superbill. In Wikipedia. Retrieved November 12, 2010 from http://en.wikipedia.org/wiki/Superbill.
[38] Fluoroscopy. In Wikipedia. Retrieved November 12, 2010 from http://en.wikipedia.org/wiki/Fluoroscopy
[39] Electromyography. In Wikipedia. Retrieved November 12,

2010 from http://en.wikipedia.org/wiki/Electromyography.
[40] Cerebrospinal_fluid. Electromyography. In Wikipedia. Retrieved November 12, 2010 from http://en.wikipedia.org/wiki/Cerebrospinal_fluid_analysis#Pathology_and_laboratory_diagnosis.
[41] Positron Emission Tomography. In Wikipedia. Retrieved November 12, 2010 from http://en.wikipedia.org/wiki/Positron_emission_tomography
[42] Physiatry. In Wikipedia. Retrieved November 12, 2010 from http://en.wikipedia.org/wiki/Physiatry.
[43] In Wikipedia. Retrieved November 12, 2010 from http://en.wikipedia.org/wiki/Proctology.
[44] Pulmonology. In Wikipedia. Retrieved November 12, 2010 from http://en.wikipedia.org/wiki/Pulmonology.
[45] Rheumatology. In Wikipedia. Retrieved November 12, 2010 from http://en.wikipedia.org/wiki/Rheumatology.
[46] Urology. In Wikipedia. Retrieved November 12, 2010 from http://en.wikipedia.org/wiki/Urology.
[47] Osteoporosis. In Wikipedia. Retrieved November 12, 2010 from http://en.wikipedia.org/wiki/Osteoporosis.
[48] Marfan Syndrome. In Wikipedia. Retrieved November 12, 2010 from http://en.wikipedia.org/wiki/Marfan_syndrome.
[49] Circulatory System. In Wikipedia. Retrieved November 12, 2010 from http://en.wikipedia.org/wiki/Circulatory_system.
[50] Angina. In Wikipedia. Retrieved November 12, 2010 from http://en.wikipedia.org/wiki/Angina.
[51] Arrythmia. In Wikipedia. Retrieved November 12, 2010 from http://en.wikipedia.org/wiki/Arrythmia.
[52] Respiratory System. In Wikipedia. Retrieved November 12, 2010 from http://en.wikipedia.org/wiki/Respiratory_system.
[53] Thoracic Diaphragm. In Wikipedia. Retrieved November 12, 2010 from http://en.wikipedia.org/wiki/Thoracic_diaphragm.
[54] Emphysema. In Wikipedia. Retrieved November 12, 2010 from http://en.wikipedia.org/wiki/Emphysema.
[55] Digestive Juices. In Wikipedia. Retrieved November 12, 2010 from http://en.wikipedia.org/wiki/Digestive_juices.
[56] Mandated Reporter. In Wikipedia. Retrieved November 12, 2010 from http://en.wikipedia.org/wiki/Mandated_reporter.
[57] Child Neglect. In Wikipedia. Retrieved November 12, 2010 from http://en.wikipedia.org/wiki/Child_neglect.

[58] Managed Care. In Wikipedia. Retrieved November 12, 2010 from http://en.wikipedia.org/wiki/Managed_care.
[59] In Wikipedia. Retrieved November 12, 2010 from http://en.wikipedia.org/wiki/Do_Not_Resuscitate.
[60] Competence. In Wikipedia. Retrieved November 12, 2010 from http://en.wikipedia.org/wiki/Competence_(law).
[61] Civil Law. In Wikipedia. Retrieved November 12, 2010 from http://en.wikipedia.org/wiki/Civil_law_(common_law).
[62] Medication Error. In Wikipedia. Retrieved November 12, 2010 from http://en.wikipedia.org/wiki/Medication_errors.
[63] Health Insurance Portability and Accountability Act. In Wikipedia. Retrieved November 12, 2010 from http://en.wikipedia.org/wiki/Health_Insurance_Portability_and_Accountability_Act.
[64] Emancipated Minor. In Wikipedia. Retrieved November 12, 2010 from http://en.wikipedia.org/wiki/Emancipated_minor.
[65] FDA. In Wikipedia. Retrieved November 12, 2010 from http://en.wikipedia.org/wiki/Fda.
[66] Diagnosis Related Group. In Wikipedia. Retrieved November 12, 2010 from http://en.wikipedia.org/wiki/Diagnosis-related_group.
[67] Accounts Receivable. In Wikipedia. Retrieved November 12, 2010 from http://en.wikipedia.org/wiki/Accounts_receivable

33 In Wikipedia. Retrieved November 12, 2010 from http://en.wikipedia.org/wiki/Accounts_receivable#Accounts_Receivable_Age_Analysis.

www.ingramcontent.com/pod-product-compliance
Lightning Source LLC
Chambersburg PA
CBHW071822080526
44589CB00012B/888